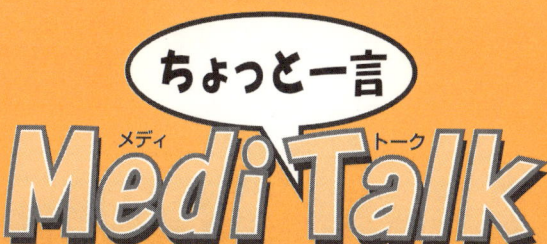

医療現場で役立つ英会話

【著　者】髙階經和・宮崎悦子
【英文監修】テレンス ジェイムズ オブライエン

インターメディカ

はじめに

　皆さんもご承知のとおり、書店には何十種類もの英会話書籍があふれています。しかし、この本は、いままでの英会話テキストや教科書とは異なったスタイルで、現場に役立つ臨床英会話を紹介しています。もし、皆さんの勤務している病院やクリニックを外国人の患者さんが訪れた場合には、医療者の方々はどう対応していますか？思わず緊張してしまう人が多いのではないでしょうか？しかし、実際に緊張しているのは、外国人の患者さんのほうなのです。外国で病気をすれば、誰でも不安な気持ちに駆られるからです。

　日本人に限らず、外国人の方にも同じことがいえます。私は50年にわたる診療経験をとおして、多くの患者さんを診てきましたが、いつも外国人の患者さんには、日本人の患者さんと同じように、ていねいに落ち着いて対応することが何よりも大切だと思っています。

　私は以前に、何冊か医学英会話の本を書いたことがあります。そして私たちは約10年前から、社団法人のボランティア活動の一環として、国際医療相談事業を行ってきました。その時、滞日中の外国人が医療機関を訪れた際、診療にはどういった日本語の会話が必要になるのかを想定して、1ページに日英対訳で双方向性の小冊子"MEDITALK"（Medical Talkingの意味で名付けました）を書きました。

　当時、この内容が各新聞や英字新聞にも紹介され、在日外国人の方々からも好評をいただきました。今回のテキストは、この小冊子の内容を参考にしながら簡単な日常会話から始め、外来診療を中心とした英会話を受付の方やナース、ドクター、コメディカルの方々のために書いたものです。

　なお、このテキストは日本語・英語の順序で書かれていますが、各Chapterでは、外国人の方々が外来にいろいろな症状で来られた際の会話を、代表的な疾患を取り上げて紹介しています。同じ人でも、その時によってわずかな表現の違いがありますので、それを、①あるいは②の文章で提示しておきました。皆さんはChapter①から始まる文章を声に出して読みながら、自分のペースで少しずつ進んでください。

　なお、このテキストにはCDが付いていますから、コンピュータやCDプレーヤーで会話を聞きながら、自分も声に出して読んでいくのが、英会話上達のもっとも効果的な方法です。では、始めてみましょう。

2004年 冬

髙階經和

C O N T

はじめに……………………………………………………… 3

Chapter 1 CALL 電話の応対に必要な英会話
- 簡単な英語を電話機の前に貼っておこう………… 8
- ちょっと一言　MediTalk……………………………… 9
- MediTalk　電話編　Call…………………………… 11

Chapter 2 OUTPATIENT 外来でよく話される英会話
- 受付の接遇が、医療機関の評判を左右します…… 16
- ちょっと一言　MediTalk……………………………… 17
- MediTalk　外来編　Outpatient…………………… 22
- 外来・受付で使われる用語………………………… 26
- 時間・カルテ用語…………………………………… 28

Chapter 3 INTERNAL MEDICINE 内科での英会話
- 病状を聞く様々な質問をしていきます…………… 32
- ちょっと一言　MediTalk……………………………… 33
- MediTalk　風邪　Cold……………………………… 43
- MediTalk　腹痛　Stomachache…………………… 48
- MediTalk　貧血　Anemia…………………………… 54
- MediTalk　糖尿病　Diabetes mellitus(Diabetes)… 59
- ちょっと一言 MediTalk　まとめ…………………… 65

Chapter 4 CARDIOLOGY 循環器科での英会話
- 高血圧などの生活習慣病がますます増えています……… 70
- ちょっと一言　MediTalk……………………………… 71
- MediTalk　高血圧
  High blood pressure(Hypertension)………… 75
- MediTalk　狭心症　Angina pectoris……………… 80
- MediTalk　高脂血症　Hyperlipidemia…………… 86
- 内科・循環器科用語………………………………… 92

Chapter 5 SURGERY ORTHOPEDICS 外科・整形外科での英会話
- 高齢の方が増え、腰痛はよく見られる症状です…100
- ちょっと一言　MediTalk………………………………101
- MediTalk　腰痛　Lumbago…………………………104
- 外科・整形外科用語…………………………………110

ENTS

PSYCHIATRY NEUROLOGY **Chapter 6** 精神・神経科での英会話
- 不眠を訴える患者さんの多様な症状に対応します……… 116
- ちょっと一言　MediTalk……………………………… 117
- MediTalk　不眠　Insomnia…………………………… 119
- 精神・神経科用語……………………………………… 125

PEDIATRICS **Chapter 7** 小児科での英会話
- 風邪やアレルギー症状が小児に多い疾患です…… 130
- ちょっと一言　MediTalk……………………………… 131
- MediTalk　小児気管支喘息
  　　　　　Child asthmatic bronchitis…………… 135
- MediTalk　小児科疾患（ヘルペス）
  　　　　　Pediatric disease (Herpes zoster)……… 140
- 小児科用語……………………………………………… 144

GYNECOLOGY **Chapter 8** 婦人科での英会話
- 不正出血は、婦人科で特に多い症状です………… 148
- ちょっと一言　MediTalk……………………………… 149
- MediTalk　不正出血　Irregular bleeding………… 151
- 産婦人科用語…………………………………………… 155

DERMATOLOGY **Chapter 9** 皮膚科での英会話
- 皮膚科の症状は非常にバラエティに富んでいます…… 160
- ちょっと一言　MediTalk……………………………… 161
- MediTalk　発疹・湿疹　Rash………………………… 163
- MediTalk　体臭　Body odor………………………… 165
- MediTalk　水虫　Athlete's foot……………………… 166
- 皮膚科用語……………………………………………… 168

- ちょっと一言　MediTalk　まとめ…………………… 169
- 系統歴…………………………………………………… 180
- 系統歴の取り方………………………………………… 183
- 体を表す用語…………………………………………… 188

著者・英文監修者プロフィール……………………………192

Chapter 1 CALL

電話の応対に必要な英会話

Just a moment, please.

One moment, please.

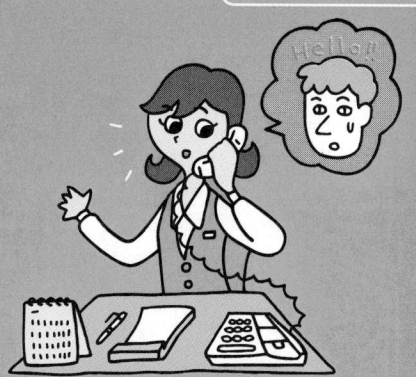

電話の応対に必要な英会話

簡単な英語を電話機の前に貼っておこう

　まず電話応対への対応策として、もし電話がかかって「Hello!」と言われたら、電話機の前の壁やボードに簡単な英語で書いてある文章、例えば「ちょっと、お待ちください」（Just a moment, please.）あるいは「少しお待ちください」（One moment, please.）を読みながら、受話器を保留にして、英語のできる人に替わってもらうのが、いちばんよい方法だと思います。

　できれば「今、先生はいらっしゃいませんが」（The doctor is not here, right now.）とか、「先生は10時に戻られます」（The doctor will be back at 10:00 am.）、あるいは「5分後にお電話いただけませんか?」（Could you call us back in 5 minutes?）といった文章もカードに書いておけば、よいかもしれませんね。ポイントは、ゆっくり話すことです。英語のできる人がだれもいない場合はお手上げですね。そんな場合に、ちょっと一言 MediTalk をご活用ください。

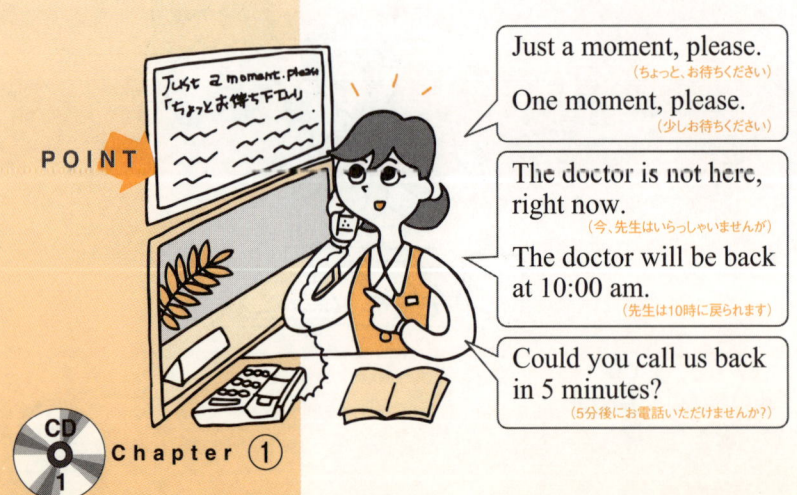

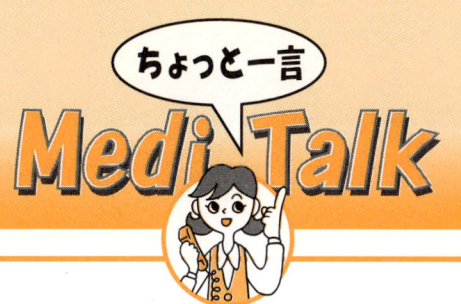

- ●もしもし、こちらは○○○クリニックです。
  Hello, this is ○○○ Clinic.

- ●日本語は話せますか？
  Do you speak Japanese?

- ●ご用件は？／どうなさいましたか？
  May I help you?

- ●診察のご予約ですか？
  Do you want to make an appointment to see a doctor?

- ●お名前をどうぞ。
  May I have your name?

- ●お電話番号を教えていただけますか？
  Would you please tell me your phone number?

- ●もう一度お願いします。
  I beg your pardon?

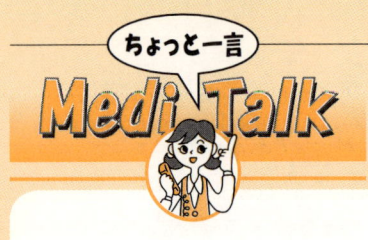

- もう一度、ゆっくり言ってください。
  Please tell me slowly again.

- あなたの予約は6月9日の午前10時です。
  You can make your appointment at 10:00 am on June 9th.

- それでよろしいですか？
  Is that okay with you?

- 保険証をお持ちでしたら、ご持参ください。
  Please bring your health insurance card, if you have one.

- あなたの診察券です。
  This is your patient ID card of this hospital (clinic).

- 当院へいらっしゃる時は、必ずこの診察券を持ってきてください。
  Whenever you come to this hospital (clinic), please bring this card.

MediTalk
電話編 / Call

Chapter 1
電話の応対に必要な英会話

では、実際に、次のような会話を想定してみましょう。
外国人の方から、田中クリニックに電話がかかってきました。

Let's think of the following conversations.
A foreigner made a call to the Tanaka Clinic.

 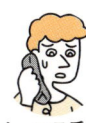
受付／斉藤

もしもし、こちらは田中クリニックです。ご用件は?

**Hello, this is Dr. Tanaka's Clinic.
May I help you?**

 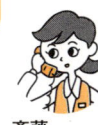
トーマス氏

もしもし、わたしはビル・トーマスと申しますが、田中先生に診ていただきたいので、予約をお願いしたいのですが。

**Hello, my name is Bill Thomas.
I would like to make an appointment to see Dr. Tanaka.**

 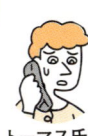
斉藤

わかりました。それでどこか具合が悪いのですか?

**I see.
And, may I ask what is wrong with you?**

 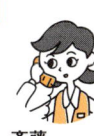
トーマス氏

ええ、3週間前から腹痛が続いているのです。できるだけ早く田中先生に診ていただきたいのです。

Well, I have had a pain in my stomach for three weeks. So, I would like to see Dr. Tanaka, as soon as possible.

5

斉藤

わかりました、トーマスさん。このクリニックはどうしてお知りになりましたか?

All right, Mr. Thomas. How did you find out about this clinic?

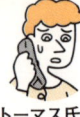

友人にこのクリニックに電話をして予約を取るように言われました。

My friend suggested that I call this clinic to make an appointment.

 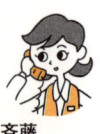

そうですか。では田中先生に診ていただきたいわけですね。

Is that right? Then, you really want to see Dr. Tanaka, right?

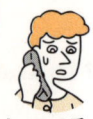

そうです。関西地方に住んでいる外国人の間で田中先生の評判が高いからです。

That is right, because Dr. Tanaka has a good reputation among foreigners living in the Kansai area.

 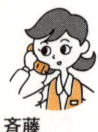

ああ、それは嬉しいです。ありがとうございます。あなたの予約は明日の午後2時に致しますが、それでよろしいですか？

Oh, I am glad to hear that, thank you. I can make your appointment at 2:00 pm tomorrow. Is that okay with you, Mr. Thomas?

 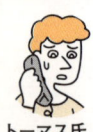

はい結構です。では明日の午後2時にそちらにまいります。

That's fine. I will be there at 2:00 pm tomorrow afternoon.

 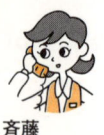

このクリニックへの地図をFAXでお送りしましょうか？

Shall I send you a map showing how to get to this clinic, by fax?

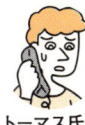

ありがとう。お願いします。

Thank you. Please do.

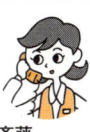

もし、おわかりにならなければ、駅の近くの公衆電話で、もう一度お電話ください。わたしの名前は斉藤といいます。

If you get lost, please call us from a public telephone near the station. My name is Ms. Saito.

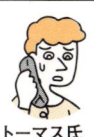

ありがとう、斉藤さん。

Thank you, Ms. Saito.

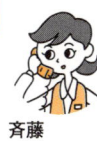

では明日、トーマスさん。もしお持ちでしたら、保険証をご持参ください。

See you tomorrow, Mr. Thomas. Please bring your health insurance card, if you have one.

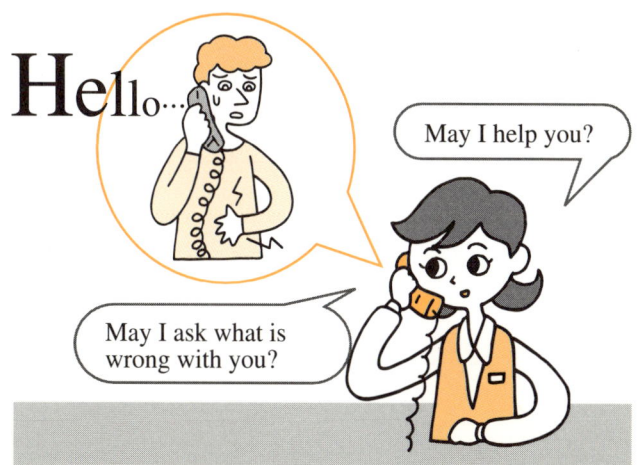

Chapter 2 OUTPATIENT

外来でよく話される英会話

How do you feel now?

Come this way, please.

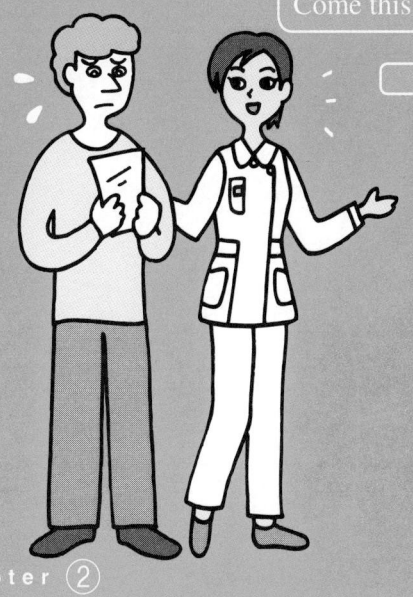

CD 1 Chapter ②

Chapter 2 OUTPATIENT

外来でよく話される英会話

受付の接遇が、医療機関の評判を左右します

　どんな病院やクリニックでも、受付の接遇態度によってその医療機関の評判をよくしたり、悪くしたりします。これは医療に限らず、どんな職業にでも言えることで、世界中どこに行っても同じことです。医療者が謙虚さを失った場合には、必ず問題が起こってくると言ってよいでしょう。

　アメリカには「全ての職業は社会に対するサービスである。そして医師もその職業の一つである」という考え方があります。これは、まさに医療者の全てにも言えることだと思います。

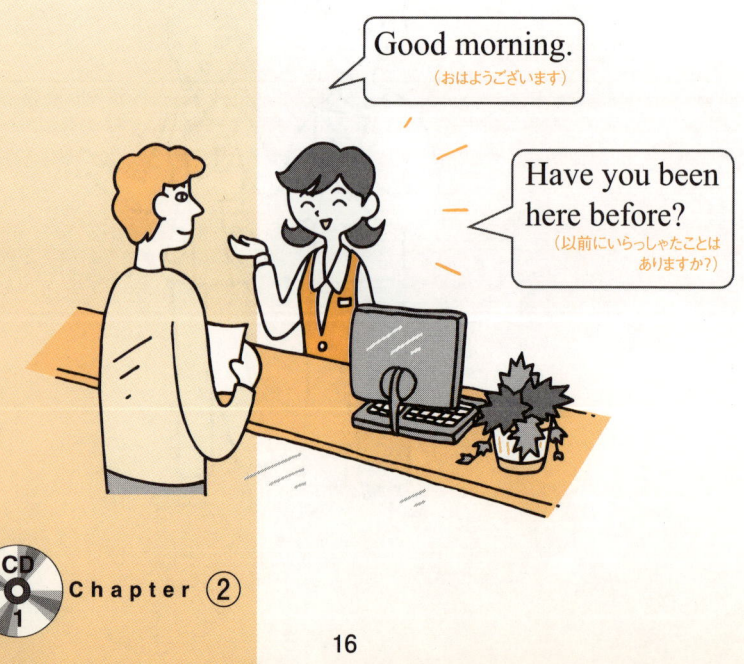

Good morning.
（おはようございます）

Have you been here before?
（以前にいらっしゃたことはありますか?）

CD1　Chapter ②

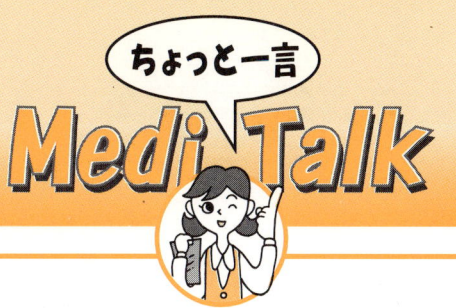

●おはようございます。
Good morning.

●お名前は？
May I have your name?

●紹介状をお持ちですか？
Do you have any reference letters?

●以前にいらっしゃったことはありますか？
Have you been here before?

●あなたのチャートを作りますので、この用紙に記入してください。
Would you fill out this form for me, so that I can make a chart for you?

●緊急時にはどなたに連絡すればよろしいですか？
In case of emergency, who shall we contact?

●何番にかければよろしいですか？
At what number?

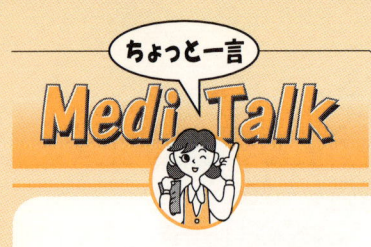

● では____番の窓口に行ってください。
Please follow the signs to counter No.____.

● これを持って____の外来に行ってください。
Please take this to the outpatient department of _____.

● 床の上の黄色い線に沿って行ってください。
Please follow the yellow line on the floor.

● このホールの突き当たりです。
It is located at the end of this hall.

● 次の角の右手にあります。
You can find it on the right at the next corner.

● すぐに総合外来の医師にあなたの症状をお話しください。
Please tell the doctor about your symptoms at the general outpatient clinic, right away.

● この病院では、約1時間は待たなければなりません。
You have to wait about one hour at this hospital.

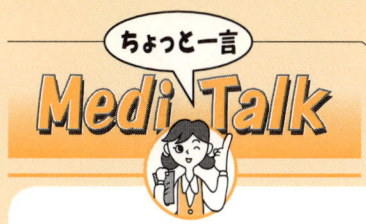

- お名前をお呼びするまで、椅子にかけてお待ちください。
  Please have a seat and wait until we call your name.

- お入りください。
  Come in, please.

- こちらへ来てください。
  Come this way, please.

- ここの椅子におかけください。
  Please have a seat here.

- どうされましたか？
  What seems to be the trouble?

- この症状で、ほかで診察をお受けになりましたか？
  Have you seen another doctor about this problem?

- 暑い（寒い）ですか？
  Do you feel hot (cold)?

- 熱はありますか？
  Do you have a fever?

- 気分はいかがですか？
  How do you feel now?

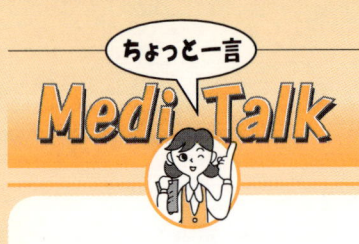

●血圧は高い方ですか？
Do you have high blood pressure?

●脈拍と血圧を測ります。
I'm going to take your pulse and blood pressure.

●アルコール類はお飲みになりますか？
Do you drink any alcohol?

●タバコはお吸いになりますか？
Do you smoke?

●先生がすぐに診てくださいます。
The doctor will see you soon.

●ご心配なく。
Don't worry.

●私に話してください。
**Tell me about it, please.
(Tell me, please.)**

●何とおっしゃいましたか？
**What did you say?
(I beg your pardon?)**

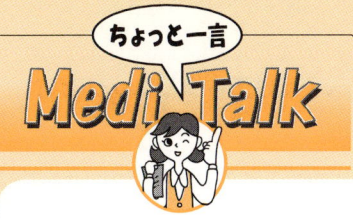

Chapter 2 外来でよく話される英会話

● すぐに戻ります。
I'll be back soon.

● ここでお待ちください。
Wait here, please.

● ちょっとお待ちください。
Just a moment, please.

● 落ち着いてください。
Calm down, please.

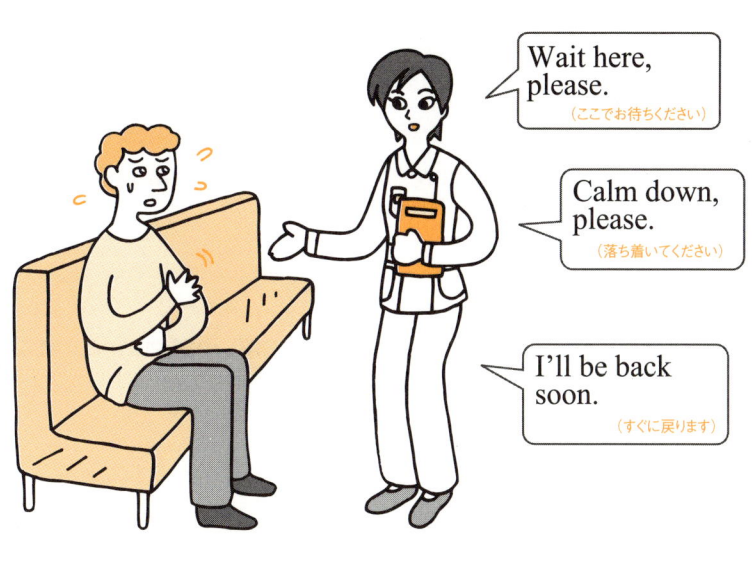

Wait here, please. (ここでお待ちください)

Calm down, please. (落ち着いてください)

I'll be back soon. (すぐに戻ります)

MediTalk
外来編 / Outpatient

翌日、午後2時、トーマスさんは田中クリニックを訪れました。

On the next day, at 2:00 pm, Mr. Thomas visited the Tanaka Clinic.

1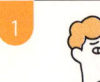
トーマス氏

やあ、わたしはビル・トーマスです。昨日予約をいたしました。

Hello, I am Bill Thomas. I made an appointment yesterday.

2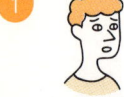
受付／斉藤

はい、トーマスさん。田中先生がすぐに診察されます。あなたのカルテをお作りしたいので、この用紙にご記入ください。

Hello, Mr. Thomas. Dr. Tanaka will see you soon. Would you fill out this form for me, so that I can make a chart for you?

3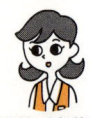
トーマス氏

（トーマス氏は、国籍、氏名、生年月日、電話番号と職業などを外来用紙に記入します）
わかりました。

Certainly.

4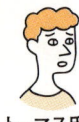
斉藤

今日は健康保険証をお持ちですか、トーマスさん？

Do you have your health insurance card today, Mr. Thomas?

5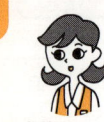
トーマス氏

いいえ、持っていません。

No, I don't have my health insurance card.

6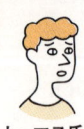
斉藤

次にいらっしゃるときに、必ず保険証を持ってきてください。

Please bring your health insurance card the next time you come.

Chapter 2 外来でよく話される英会話

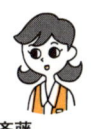
トーマス氏

はい、必ず持ってきます。
Yes, I'll certainly bring it the next time.

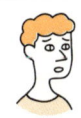
斉藤

保険証がなければ、今日は自費になりますが、よろしいですか?
If you don't have the health insurance card today, you have to pay the full medical bill. Is that OK?

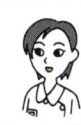
トーマス氏

ええ、結構です。
Yes, I'll pay it.

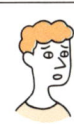
ナース／石田

トーマスさん、どうぞお入りください。
Mr. Thomas, won't you come in please?

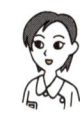
トーマス氏

(トーマス氏は診察室に入ってきます)
はい。わたしはビル・トーマスです。
Yes.
I am Bill Thomas.

石田

(ドクター田中が診察室に入って来る前に、少し質問をしています)
わたしは看護師の石田です。このクリニックへはどうしていらしたのですか?
I am Nurse Ishida. What brings you to this clinic?

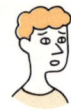
トーマス氏

昨日も斉藤さんに電話でお話ししたのですが、3週間も腹痛が続いています。それで田中先生に今日診ていただこうと決めたのです。

As I told Ms. Saito on the telephone yesterday, I have had an abdominal pain for three weeks. So, I have decided to see Dr. Tanaka today.

 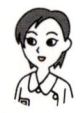
石田

そうですか。このクリニックにいらっしゃる前に、ほかの先生に診ていただきましたか?

Is that right? Did you see any other doctor, before coming to this clinic?

 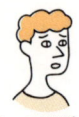
トーマス氏

いいえ、診てもらっていません。

No, I did not.

 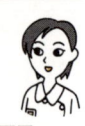
石田

家で体温を測りましたか?

Did you check your temperature at home?

 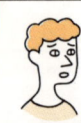
トーマス氏

ええ、測りました。しかし、毎日ではありません。

Yes, I did. But, I do not it everyday.

 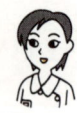
石田

(体温を測ります)
体温をお測りしましょう。口を開けてこの体温計を1分間、舌の下に入れてください。

Let's take your temperature. Please keep this thermometer under your tongue for one minute.

 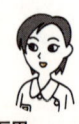
石田

おやっ、少しお熱がありますね。

Well, you have a slight fever.

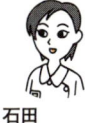
石田

（脈を測ります）
脈をとりましょう。右腕を出してください。

I'd like to take your pulse now. Please hold out your right arm.

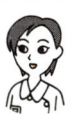
石田

（血圧を測ります）
血圧をお測りしましょう。左腕の袖をまくってください。そしてこの台の上に乗せ、リラックスしてください。

I'd like to check your blood pressure. Please roll up your left sleeve, rest your arm on this pad, and try to relax.

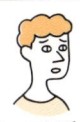
トーマス氏

わたしの血圧はどうですか？　正常ですか？

How is my blood pressure? Is it all right?

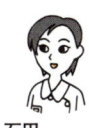
石田

血圧は130/80mmHgで、正常です。

Your blood pressure is 130/80mmHg, and this is normal.

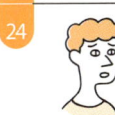
トーマス氏

それを聞いて安心しました。血圧が高いのではないかと心配していましたから。

I am glad to hear that. I was worrying if my blood pressure might be high.

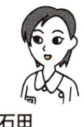
石田

もうすぐ田中先生がいらっしゃいますから、お待ちください。

Dr. Tanaka will be here soon. Please wait for a minute.

外来・受付で使われる用語

あ

医学生	medical student
医師	physician, medical doctor
受付 / 受付係	reception / receptionist
栄養士	dietician

か

科、部	department, unit
会計	cashier
回復室	recovery room
外来	OPD (outpatient department)
眼科	ophthalmology department
看護師詰所	nurses' station
看護助手	nurse's aid
看護部長	superintendent of nurses, matron (British only)
冠疾患集中管理室	CCU (coronary care unit)
機能訓練室	rehabilitation room
救急病棟	emergency ward
外科	surgical department, dept. of surgery
結核病棟	tuberculosis ward
検査室	laboratory
個室	private room

さ

産科	obstetric department
歯科	dental department
耳鼻咽喉科	ear, nose and throat department
集中治療室	ICU (intensive care unit)
手術室	OR (operating room)
主任（看護師）	head nurse
小児科	pediatric department
食堂	dining room
処置室	treatment room
神経外科	neuro-surgical department
診察室	examining room, consultation room

	水療法室	hydrotherapy room
	正看護師	registered nurse
	整形外科	orthopedic department
	精神科	psychiatric department
	総合病院	general hospital
た	中央材料室	central supply
	電気療法室	electrotherapy room
	伝染病棟	contagious/communicable disease ward
	当直医	doctors on duty
な	内科	medical department, internal medicine
	熱傷集中管理室	burn care unit (BCU)
は	非常出口	fire escape
	皮膚科	dermatology department
	病室（棟）	ward
	部、科	department, unit
	婦人科	gynecology department
	分娩室	delivery room
ま	待合室	waiting room
や	薬剤師	pharmacist
	薬局	pharmacy
ら	レントゲン室	X-ray room

時間・カルテ用語

あ

朝	morning
明後日	the day after tomorrow
明日	tomorrow
一昨日	the day before yesterday
温度表	graphic sheet, TPR sheet

か

外来患者	outpatient
カルテ	chart
昨日	yesterday
今日	today
記録	recording
経過用紙	progress sheet
検査報告用紙	laboratory report sheet
検査要求用紙	laboratory request sheet
午後	afternoon
今月	this month

さ

時間	hour
指示用紙	order sheet
疾病	disease, illness, sickness
承諾書、同意書	consent form
診断	diagnosis
請求書	bill
先週	last week

た

第1日目	the first day
退院	discharge
退院届け	discharge notice
月	month
転室届け	transfer notice
同意書／承諾書	consent form/ agreement form
時	time

な		
	入院	admission
	入院患者	inpatient
	入院届け	admission notice
	入院日数	hospital day, admission day
	入院用紙	admission sheet
	年	year

は		
	日	day
	日付	date
	秒	second
	病歴	history
	病歴用紙	history sheet
	昼	noon
	分	minute
	保険用紙	insurance paper

ま		
	3日前	three days ago

や		
	夕方	evening
	用紙	form, record sheet
	夜	night

ら		
	領収証	receipt

Chapter 3 INTERNAL MEDICINE

内科での英会話

Can I help you?

Do you feel tired?

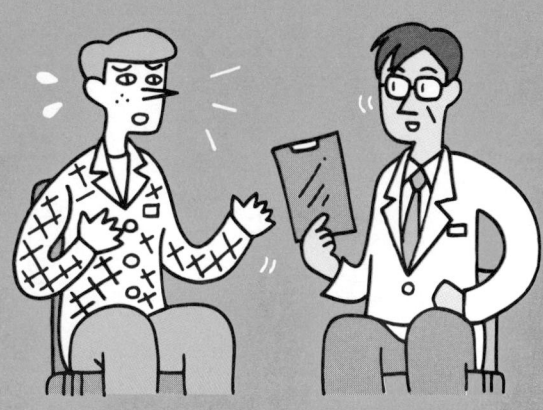

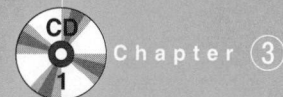
Chapter ③

Chapter 3
INTERNAL MEDICINE
内科での英会話

病状を聞く様々な質問をしていきます

どんな病気でも、まず症状が出ると患者さんは一般内科や総合外来を受診することがほとんどですね。

病院や医療機関によっても違いがありますが、最初に病状を聞くのはナースの方々だと思います。どうして来られたのか、具合の悪いのはどこか、いつから悪いのか、どうしてそうなったのか、今までお医者さんにかかったことはないかなど、様々な質問が考えられます。

では、実際にどんなことを聞いていくのかをみていきましょう。

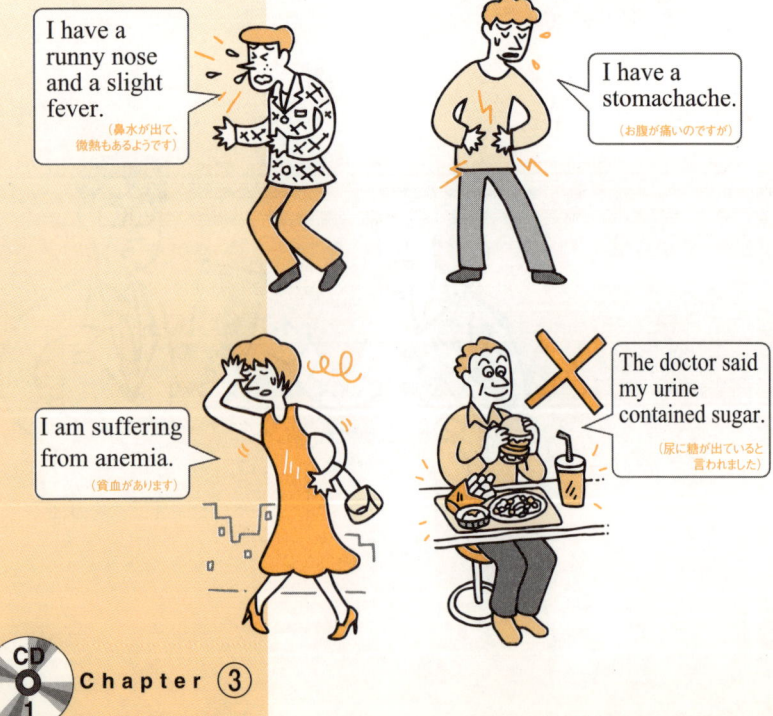

I have a runny nose and a slight fever.
（鼻水が出て、微熱もあるようです）

I have a stomachache.
（お腹が痛いのですが）

I am suffering from anemia.
（貧血があります）

The doctor said my urine contained sugar.
（尿に糖が出ていると言われました）

CD 1 Chapter 3

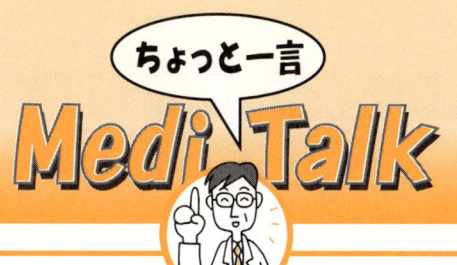

● 英語が得意ではありませんので、ゆっくりお話しください。
I speak very little English, so please speak slowly.

● 「はい」か「いいえ」で答えていただけますか。
When possible, answer with "yes" or "no".

● どうなさいましたか？
Can I help you?

● いつからですか？
Since when?

● 時々頭痛がしますか？
Do you have frequent headaches?

● 頭痛はどんな種類のものですか？
What's kind of headache you have?

● お医者さんに行きましたか？
Did you see a doctor?

● 頭痛の時は何か薬を飲みますか？
Do you take any medicine for your headache?

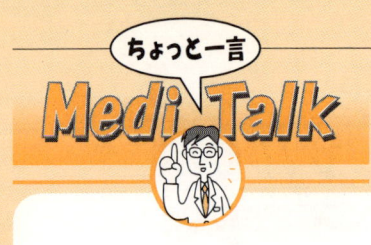

●いつもどんな薬で頭痛がなくなりますか？
What kind of medicine do you usually take to relieve your headache?

●今まで、あるいは最近、視力が変わったことに気付きましたか？
Have you noticed any change in your vision in the past or lately?

●まぶたの炎症や、腫れを起こしたことはありますか？
Did you have any inflammation or swelling in your eyelids?

●眼鏡なしでよく見えますか？
Can you see well without glasses?

●目が痛くなったことがありますか？　友人から眼球が突出しているとか、陥没しているとか言われたことはありますか？
Have you noticed any pain in your eyes, or has anyone said that your eyes are bulging out, or sunken?

●聴力はよい方ですか？
Do you have good hearing?

●耳鳴りに気付いたことがありますか？
Have you noticed any ringing in your ears?

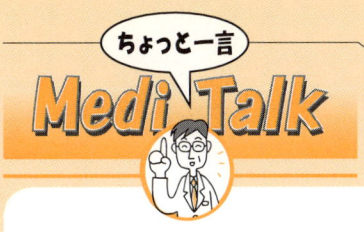

●めまいを起こしたことはありますか？
Do you ever feel dizzy (vertigo)?

●外耳道から分泌物が出たことがありますか？
Have you ever had any discharge from your ear canal?

●鼻腔の後ろの方に鼻汁が出たり、鼻が詰まったりしますか？
Do you have a postnasal drip or stopped-up nose?

●時々鼻血が出ますか？
Do you have frequent nose bleeds?

●よく風邪をひきますか？
Do you catch cold quite often?

●激しい咳がありますか？
Do you have a severe cough?

●いつ頃から咳が出始めましたか？
How long have you had the cough?

●痰が出ますか？
Do you have any phlegm?

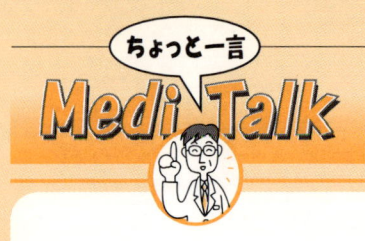

●どんな色の痰が出ますか？　黄色、透明、白、緑っぽいですか？
What color is it?
Is it yellow, clear, white or green?

●喉の痛みがありますか？
Do you have a sore throat?

●つばを飲み込むと痛いですか？
Does it hurt when you swallow?

●どのくらい痛みが続いていますか？
How long have you had this pain?

> 3〜4時間
> **for three or four hours**
>
> 1週間ほど
> **for about a week**
>
> 昨夜から
> **since last night**

●口唇や口腔内に潰瘍ができたことがありますか？
Have you ever had any ulcers on your lips, or inside your mouth?

●歯の具合はどうですか？
How are your teeth?

ちょっと一言 Medi Talk

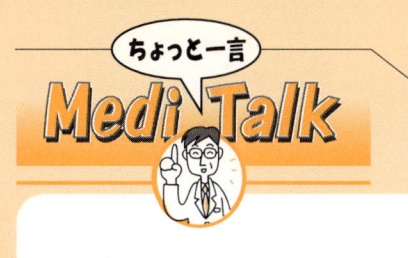

Chapter 3 内科での英会話

●扁桃腺は取りましたか？
Have you had your tonsils out?

●今までに食物を飲み込みにくくなったことがありますか？
Have you ever had any difficulty in swallowing?

●症状が起きたのはいつですか？
When did this happen to you?

   3日前
   three days ago
   4週間前
   four weeks ago

●タバコはお吸いになりますか？
Do you smoke cigarettes?

●1日にどのくらい吸いますか？
How many per day?

●1日1箱ですか？
One pack a day?

●それ以上ですか？
More?

Medi Talk ちょっと一言

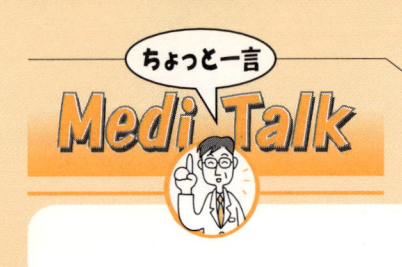

●それ以下ですか？
Less?

●結核になったことはありますか？
Have you had tuberculosis?

●喘息になったことはありますか？
Have you had asthma?

●今までに薬のアレルギーがありましたか？
Have you ever had an allergy to medication?

●今までに、薬で副作用が出たことがありますか？
Have you ever had any side effects from your medicine?

●今はどこが痛みますか？
Where is the pain now?

●指で痛むところを指してください。
Please point to it with your finger.

●食欲はありますか？
Do you have a good appetite?

●体がだるいですか？
Do you feel tired?

ちょっと一言 Medi Talk

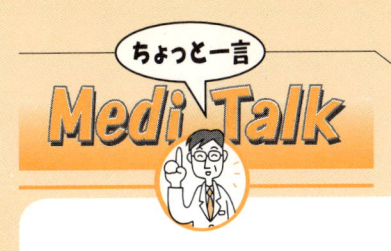

●食事をすると痛みがひどくなりますか？
Does eating make the pain worse?

●食事をとらなくても痛みますか？
Do you feel pain without eating?

●食べる前（後）によく起こりますか？
Does your pain occur more frequently before (after) meals?

●油っぽいものを食べると痛みがひどくなりますか？
Does greasy food make the pain worse?

●痛みが楽になる姿勢はありますか？
Is there any position that makes the pain better?

●横になりますか？　前屈みはどうですか？
Lying down? Bending forward?

●便通はいかがですか？
How about your bowel movement?

下痢
diarrhea

便秘
constipation

ちょっと一言 Medi Talk

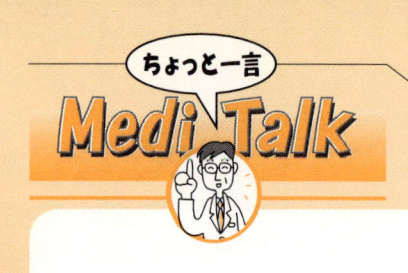

●血便はなかったですか？
Have you noticed blood in your stools, or in the toilet?

●タールのように黒い便は出ませんか？
Are your stools black like tar?

●手術を受けたことはありますか？
Have you had any operations?

> 虫垂炎
> for an appendix
> 胆石
> for gallstones

●潰瘍になったことはありますか？
Have you had an ulcer?

●今までに胃の検査を受けたことがありますか？
Have you ever had a stomach examination?

●腹部エコー検査を受けたことがありますか？
Have you had an abdominal echogram test?

ちょっと一言 Medi Talk

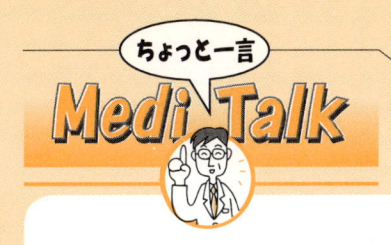

Chapter 3 内科での英会話

●胃薬を飲んでいますか？
Do you take medicine for your stomach?

●息切れしますか？
Do you have shortness of breath?

●疲労感が強いですか？
Do you feel much tired?

●よく眠れますか？
Do you sleep well?

●胸痛はありますか？
Do you have any chest pain?

●下肢にむくみはありますか？
Do you have any edema in your legs?

●以前にも貧血がありましたか？
Have you ever suffered from anemia?

●潰瘍があると言われたことはありますか？
Has it ever been pointed out to you that you had an ulcer?

Medi Talk
ちょっと一言

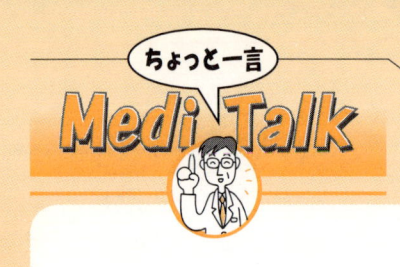

●大便に血が混ざったことがありますか？
Have you had any blood in your stools?

●いつもどんなお薬を飲んでいますか？
What kind of medicine do you usually take?

抗うつ薬
antidepressant

睡眠薬
sleeping pills

ビタミン剤
vitamin tablets

●何かお薬(サプリメント)を服用されていますか？
Are you taking any medicines (supplements) now?

MediTalk

風邪 / Cold

Chapter 3 — 内科での英会話

スミスさんが田中クリニックを訪れました。

Mr. Smith visited the Tanaka Clinic.

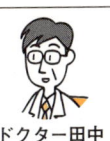

---

1. ドクター田中

どうしましたか?

① What seems to be the trouble?

② What can I do for you today?

---

2. スミス氏

鼻水が出て、微熱もあるようです。

I have a runny nose and a slight fever.

---

3. ドクター田中

いつ頃からですか?

① How long have you had it?

② When did it start?

---

4. スミス氏

2日前からです。

① It started two days ago.

② It's been bothering me for two days now.

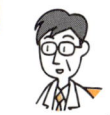

---

5. ドクター田中

熱はどのくらい出ましたか? それはいつですか?

How high has your temperature been, and when did you have a fever?

---

6. スミス氏

昨日の夕方、だるかったので測ったら37.5℃ありました。

① Because I felt so weak, I took my temperature last night, and it was 37.5°C.

② Last night I felt weak, so I took my temperature and it was 37.5°C.

7 ドクター田中

ほかに何か症状がありますか?

① Do you have any other symptoms?

② Is there anything else bothering you?

8 スミス氏

喉が痛いのです。

① I also have a sore throat.

② Yes, my throat hurts, too.

9 ドクター田中

食事をする時、痛みますか?

① Does your throat hurt when you eat?

② Is it painful when you eat?

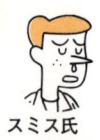

10 スミス氏

食べ物を飲み込む時、痛みます。

It hurts each time I swallow.

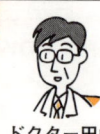

11 ドクター田中

咳をすると痰が出ますか?

Have you been coughing up phlegm?

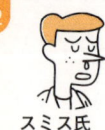

12 スミス氏

少しです。

A little.

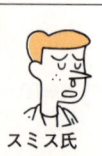

13 スミス氏

いまのところ空咳だけです。

No, it's been basically a dry cough so far.

Chapter 3　内科での英会話

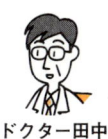

14 ドクター田中
血痰に気付いたことがありますか？
Have you ever noticed any blood in the phlegm?

15 スミス氏
はい、今朝気付きました。
Yes, I noticed it this morning.

16 ドクター田中
タバコを吸いますか？
Do you smoke?

17 スミス氏
はい。
Yes.

18 スミス氏
1日に1箱ぐらい吸います。
I smoke one pack a day.

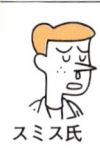

19 スミス氏
①どうしても、やめられないので。
I just can't stop smoking.

②いいえ。全く吸ったことがありません。
No, I do not smoke at all.

③数年前にやめました。
I stopped smoking a few years ago.

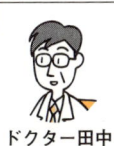

20 ドクター田中
食欲はいかがですか？
How has your appetite been?

| 21 | スミス氏 | あまりありません。 |

① I've lost my appetite, unfortunately.

② I haven't had much of an interest in eating lately.

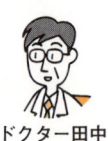

| 22 | ドクター田中 | 便通の具合は変わりましたか？ 回数は1日どのくらいですか？ |

Have there been any changes in your stool? How many times do you have a bowel movement a day?

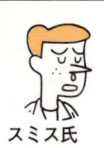

| 23 | スミス氏 | 多少、便がゆるいようです。しかし、そんなに多くはありません。 |

I have a loose stool, but I haven't had to go to the bathroom so many times each day.

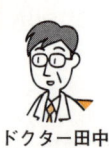

| 24 | ドクター田中 | 尿が濁ったり、排尿の時に痛かったりしませんか？ |

① Is your urine cloudy? Do you feel pain when you urinate?

② Have you noticed if your urine has become cloudy? Is there any pain which accompanies urination?

| 25 | スミス氏 | 排尿した後、痛みます。 |

① I've been having pain after I urinate.

② There has been some pain which comes after urination.

| 26 | ドクター田中 | ご家族や職場の方で、風邪をひいている人はいますか？ |

① Is there anyone in your family or at work who has a cold now?

② Have you been around anyone at home or at work who also has a cold?

---

27 スミス氏

幼稚園に行っている子供が風邪をひいています。

① My child, who goes to kindergarten, has been suffering from a cold.

② Yes, my kindergarten-age child has had a cold.

---

28 ドクター田中

では、ちょっと診てみましょう。口を大きく開けてください。

I'd like to examine you now. Open your mouth wide.

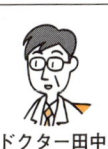

---

29 ドクター田中

喉が赤くなっていて、扁桃腺が腫れていますね。

① Your throat looks red, and your tonsils are swollen.

② I can see some inflammation in your throat as well as swelling in your tonsils.

---

30 ドクター田中

リンパ腺を調べましょう。呼吸音を聞きますから胸を開けてください。

I'll check for swelling in your lymph nodes now. I'd like to listen to your respiration, so please lift up (open) your shirt.

---

31 ドクター田中

呼吸音に異常はないようです。

① There seems to be no problem with your breathing.

② Your breathing sounds clear, so there's no problem there.

MediTalk

腹痛
Stomachache

トーマスさんが今朝、田中クリニックを再診で訪れました。

Mr. Thomas revisited the Tanaka Clinic this morning.

---

1 ドクター田中

こんにちは、トーマスさん。その後、どうしておられましたか？今日はどうなさいましたか？

Hello, Mr. Thomas. How have you been?

① What can I do for you today?

② What seems to be the trouble with you today?

---

2 トーマス氏

お腹が痛いのですが。

① I have a stomachache.

② My stomach hurts.

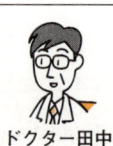

---

3 ドクター田中

どんな痛みで、どのくらい続いていますか？

① What kind of pain is it, and how long have you had it?

② Can you describe the pain, and tell me when it started?

---

4 トーマス氏

鈍くとぎれとぎれの痛みで、1週間ぐらい断続的に続いています。

① It's a dull, intermittent pain. I've had it for about a week now, off and on.

② The pain is a dull ache that comes and goes. I first felt it about a week ago.

5 ドクター田中

特にどんなときに痛みますか？

① When do you feel the pain particularly?

② When does it usually hurt?

6 トーマス氏

空腹時に特に強く痛みます。

① It's especially strong when I'm hungry.

② It seems to hit me whenever I'm hungry.

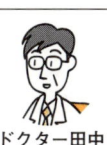

7 ドクター田中

何かほかに症状がありますか？

① Do you have any other symptoms?

② Have you experienced any other symptoms recently?

8 トーマス氏

ええ、時々胸焼けがします。それから最近2キロもやせました。

① Yes, I sometimes have heartburn. And I've lost 2kg recently.

② As a matter of fact, yes. I've lost 2kg, and every once in a while I have occasional heartburn.

9 ドクター田中

それはいけませんね。

Is that right?

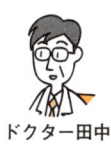

10 ドクター田中

今までに何か大きな病気をしたことがありますか？

Have you had any serious illnesses before?

Chapter 3 内科での英会話

11 トーマス氏

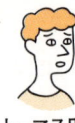

いいえ、ありません。

Never, Doctor.

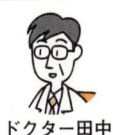

---

12 ドクター田中

仕事はいかがですか？　前よりも忙しいですか？

① How's your work going? Are you busier than you were before?

② Tell me about your work. For example, has it gotten busier lately?

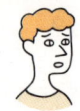

---

13 トーマス氏

ええ、仕事はうまくいっていますが、先月ゼネラルマネージャーに昇進したこともあって、かなり忙しく、毎日2時間以上残業しています。

Yes, you are right. Since being promoted to general manager last month, I've averaged two hours of overtime everyday.

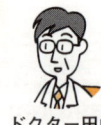

---

14 ドクター田中

それは大変ですね。ところで、タバコは吸いますか？

① That's too bad. By the way, do you smoke?

② Sounds tough. Tell me, are you a smoker?

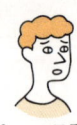

---

15 トーマス氏

はい、よくないことですが、1日平均1箱ほど吸います。

① Unfortunately, yes. I average a pack of cigarettes a day.

② I hate to admit it, but I average a pack of cigarettes a day.

Chapter 3

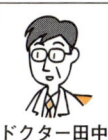

16 ドクター田中

お酒はどうですか？
What about drinking?

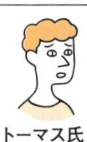

17 トーマス氏

夕食時にビール1本ほど飲みます。
I usually have a bottle of beer at dinner.

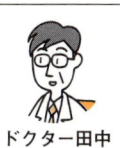

18 ドクター田中

それではちょっと診察してみましょう。シャツを脱いでいただけますか。

① **Okay, I'd like to examine you now. Please take off your shirt.**

② **Okay. Let's have a look at you. Would you mind removing your shirt?**

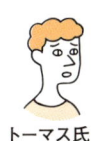

19 トーマス氏

わかりました、先生。
All right, Doctor.

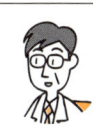

20 ドクター田中

（診察をすませたドクター田中は、石田さんに検査を指示します）
石田さん、トーマスさんの血液検査と腹部レントゲン写真を撮る指示箋を書いてください。

Ms. Ishida, please write the order sheet for Mr. Thomas, to have a blood test and abdominal X-ray films.

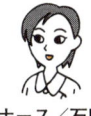

21 ナース／石田

わかりました、先生。
Yes, Doctor.

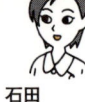

22 石田 (トーマス氏に対して)
血液検査をしますから、左腕をまくっていただけますか?
ちょっと痛いかもしれませんが、すぐに終わりますから、少しの間、ご辛抱ください。

We'll do a blood test now. Could you roll up your left sleeve? It might be a little painful, but it'll soon be over, so please be patient.

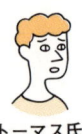

23 トーマス氏 ご心配なく。わたしは男ですよ。

Don't worry about it. I am a man.

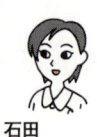

24 石田 では、腹部のレントゲンを撮ります。レントゲン室までご案内しましょう。

It's necessary for us to take an abdominal X-ray. I'll show you to the X-ray room.

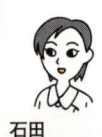

25 石田 ここの検査が終わったら腹部エコー検査をいたしますので、ここでお待ちください。

After this test, we'll do an abdominal echo-test. So, please wait here.

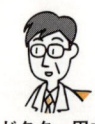

26 ドクター田中 (再び、診察室に戻ったトーマス氏に、ドクター田中が説明しています)
この錠剤を1錠ずつ1日3回飲んでください。そして、1週間後の同じ時間に来てください。

Take one of these tablets three times a day, and come back to see me a week from today at the same time.

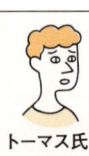

27 トーマス氏 はい。わかりました。

Okay. I've got it.

Chapter 3 内科での英会話

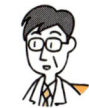

28 ドクター田中
胃の検査を行いますので、前の晩から食事や水分は控えてください。

I'll run some tests on your stomach, so be sure to refrain from eating or drinking anything from the night before.

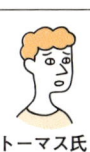

---

29 トーマス氏
わかりました。ところでこれは重い病気でしょうか?

① Okay. Do you think it's anything serious?

② Okay. Do I have anything to worry about?

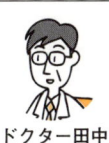

---

30 ドクター田中
今までの検査では、そうは思いません。でも、タバコやお酒は控えめにしてください。

① No, I don't think so, from the results of the tests. But you should cut down on your smoking and drinking, anyway.

② No. If I were you, I wouldn't be too concerned, but I would reduce or stop altogether the smoking and drinking.

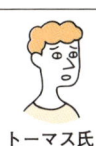

---

31 トーマス氏
わかりました、先生。どうもありがとうございました。

① Yes, Doctor. I understand. Thank you very much.

② I see what you mean, Doctor. Thanks a lot.

---

32 ドクター田中
どういたしまして。それではまた来週。

① You're welcome. See you next week.

② My pleasure. I'll be looking for you next week.

MediTalk

貧血
Anemia

アンダーソンさんが田中クリニックを訪れました。

Ms. Anderson visited the Tanaka Clinic.

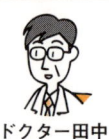

---

1 ドクター田中

どうなさいました?

What seems to be the trouble?

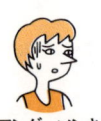

---

2 アンダーソンさん

健康診断で貧血があると言われました。最近、歩いていて動悸、息切れがします。

When I had a physical examination recently, the doctor said that I was suffering from anemia. Also, I've had palpitations and problems with catching my breath while walking.

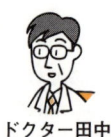

---

3 ドクター田中

白血球数、血小板数は測りましたか?

① **Did he check how many white blood corpuscles or blood platelets you have?**

② **Did he get counts of your white blood corpuscles and blood platelets?**

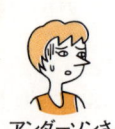

---

4 アンダーソンさん

少し少ない、と聞いています。

① **Yes, he said the numbers were low.**

② **Yes, he told me they were below normal.**

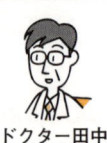

---

5 ドクター田中

熱はありますか?

Have you had a fever?

6 アンダーソンさん

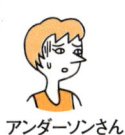

いいえ。
No, I haven't.

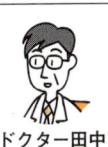

7 ドクター田中

歯肉出血や紫斑などがありますか？
Do you have any bleeding from your gums or purple spots on your skin?

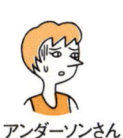

8 アンダーソンさん

いいえ。
No, I don't.

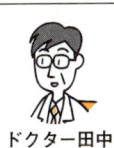

9 ドクター田中

健康診断で黄疸があると言われましたか？
① Did the doctor say that you were suffering from jaundice?
② Did the doctor mention the possibility of jaundice?

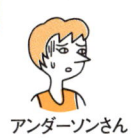

10 アンダーソンさん

健康診断では検査していないようです。
① It was never mentioned in the physical examination.
② No, he never made a reference to that.

11 ドクター田中

今まで胃腸の病気をしましたか？
① Have you ever had any stomach or intestinal illnesses?
② Have you ever suffered from stomach or intestinal problems?

12 アンダーソンさん

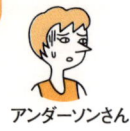

胃潰瘍で抗潰瘍剤を服用していたことがあります。

① I used to take antiulcer drugs for a gastric ulcer.

② Yes, I was treated for a gastric ulcer with antiulcer drugs.

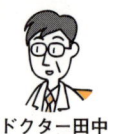

13 ドクター田中

便の色が黒くなったことがありますか?

Has your stool ever become black?

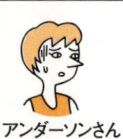

14 アンダーソンさん

気が付いたことはありません。

No, not that I've been aware of.

15 ドクター田中

まず、貧血の検査と白血球数、血小板数を測定しましょう。

First of all, I need to check the type of your anemia, so I'll get a count of your white blood corpuscles and blood platelets.

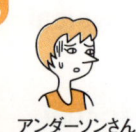

16 アンダーソンさん

わかりました、先生。

Okay, Doctor.

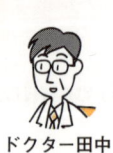

17 ドクター田中

貧血が出る病気の中には、例えば、白血球が増えたり、血小板が減る病気があります。

Many types of diseases cause anemia. For example, the disease of increasing white blood corpuscles, and decreasing blood platelets.

| 18 | アンダーソンさん | はい、わかりました。
Yes, I understand. |

| 19 | ドクター田中 | また、貧血で、黄疸が出ることがあります。これには、血清中のビリルビンを測定することが必要です。
And, a type of anemia causes jaundice, so it'll be necessary to examine the bilirubin in your serum. |

| 20 | アンダーソンさん | わかりました。
Okay. |

| 21 | ドクター田中 | また貧血の原因の一つとして、胃腸からの出血によることがあります。便の潜血反応を見ましょう。また、血清中の鉄が不足しているか、検査しましょう。
Also, bleeding from the stomach and intestines is one of the causes of anemia. We'll need to take an occult blood test of your stool, and also we need a test to see if you have enough iron in your serum. |

| 22 | ドクター田中 | （2日後にアンダーソンさんは田中クリニックを訪れます）
鉄欠乏性貧血があります。胃潰瘍はどのような状態か主治医から聞いていますか？
① **I think you're suffering from iron deficiency anemia. Did you hear from your doctor about how your gastric ulcer was?**
② **Your condition appears to be iron deficiency anemia. Did your doctor check the status of your gastric ulcer?** |

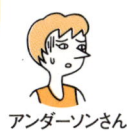

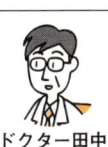

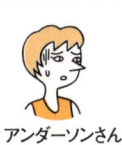

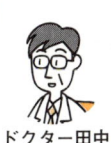

23 アンダーソンさん

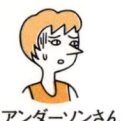

治ったことを胃カメラで確認していただきました。

He checked to make sure it was healed by using a gastro camera.

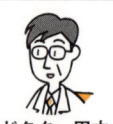

24 ドクター田中

便の潜血反応が陽性なので、ファイバースコープで大腸検査をしてみましょう。

① **The occult blood test of your stool was positive, so we'll have to examine your large intestine by fiberscope.**

② **I'd like to take a closer look at your large intestine by fiberscope, since the result of the occult blood test of your stool was positive.**

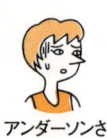

25 アンダーソンさん

はい。

All right.

26 ドクター田中

それから、血小板数6万/μl、白血球数3,500/μl とやや低いので骨髄穿刺で骨髄をみておく必要があります。

Your blood platelets are 60,000/μl, and your white blood corpuscles are 3,500/μl. These figures are rather low, so it's necessary to examine your bone marrow by bone marrow puncture.

Chapter 3 内科での英会話

MediTalk

糖尿病
Diabetes mellitus (Diabetes)

ヘイルさんが、会社の健康診断で異常を指摘され、田中クリニックを訪れました。

Mr. Hale visited the Tanaka Clinic, because he had some abnormal results from a routine physical check-up at his company.

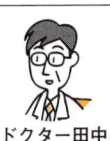

---

1 ドクター田中

どうしました？

What can I do for you today?

---

2 ヘイル氏

先日、健康診断で尿に糖が出ていると言われました。

When I had a physical examination recently, the doctor said my urine contained sugar.

---

3 ドクター田中

血糖は測りましたか？

① **Did he check your blood sugar?**

② **Did he get a blood sugar count?**

---

4 ヘイル氏

朝食前の血糖が120mg/dlあると言われました。

Yes. He said it was 120mg/dl before breakfast.

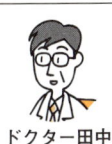

---

5 ドクター田中

尿に蛋白は出ていましたか？

① **Was there any protein in your urine?**

② **Did any protein show up in your urine?**

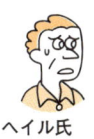

---

6 ヘイル氏

いいえ。

No.

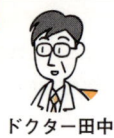

7 ドクター田中
眼底検査は受けましたか?
Did you take an eye ground test?

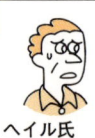

8 ヘイル氏
いいえ、受けていません。
No, I didn't.

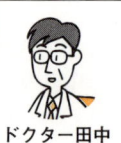

9 ドクター田中
ご家族の中で糖尿病の方はいらっしゃいますか?
① **Have any family members suffered from diabetes mellitus?**
② **Has there been any incidence of diabetes mellitus in your family?**

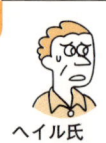

10 ヘイル氏
母親が糖尿病のため失明して、現在、血液透析を受けています。
① **My mother went blind from diabetes mellitus, and she's undergoing hemodialysis now.**
② **Yes, it caused my mother to go blind. She's being treated by hemodialysis now.**

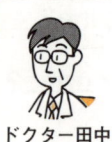

11 ドクター田中
お母さんは、どんな治療を受けておられましたか?
What kind of medical treatment did your mother used to receive?

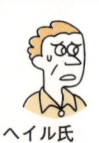

12 ヘイル氏
インスリン注射をしていました。
She used to take insulin shots.

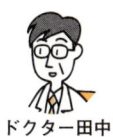

13 ドクター田中
ところで、今まで何か大きな病気をしたことがありますか?
By the way, have you ever had any serious illnesses?

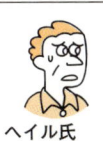

14 ヘイル氏
特にありません。
No, I haven't, Doctor.

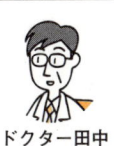

15 ドクター田中
自覚症状はありますか? 例えば、喉が渇くとか、手洗いに何度も行くとか、体重が減るとか、食欲がないとか、だるくて疲れやすいとか、あるいはスタミナがなくなり、体が重く体力が衰えたとか?
Have you had any symptoms such as a heavy thirst, frequent urination, weight loss, loss of appetite, or a dull, run-down feeling accompanied by a lack of stamina?

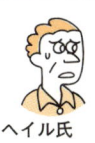

16 ヘイル氏
そう言われれば、1年間で体重が6キロも減り、夜も時々手洗いに行くことがあります。
Actually, I've lost 6kg in the past year, and I sometimes go to the bathroom at night.

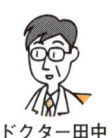

17 ドクター田中
体に化膿しやすいところとか、かゆいところはありませんか?
Do you have any skin infections filled with pus, or itching on your body?

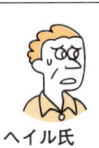

18 ヘイル氏
ありません。
Nothing.

19 ドクター田中

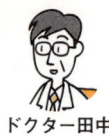

新聞の小さな字が読めますか？　脚や手のしびれや痛みはありませんか？　歯槽膿漏や歯が抜けやすいことはありませんか？

Can you read the small print in a newspaper? Do you feel numbness or pain in your legs or your hands? Have you been suffering from alveolar pyorrhea or do your teeth seem to be getting loose?

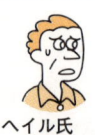

20 ヘイル氏

夜寝ている時に両足にしびれを感じたことがあります。

I have felt numbness in my feet while sleeping.

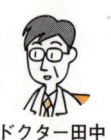

21 ドクター田中

身長と現在の体重を教えてください。

Please give me your height and present weight.

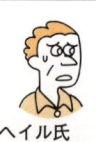

22 ヘイル氏

175センチ、76キロです。

① 175cm, and 76kg.

② I'm 175cm tall, and weigh 76kg.

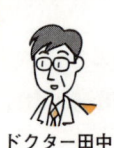

23 ドクター田中

30歳頃、いちばん太っていた時、一番やせていた時の体重はどのくらいありましたか？

How much did you weigh when you were around 30 years old, from the heaviest you can remember, to the lightest?

Chapter 3 — 内科での英会話

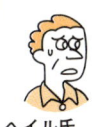

24 ヘイル氏

30歳頃の体重は70キロで、入社してから急に体重が増え90キロもあったことがありました。大学1年の頃は60キロしかありませんでした。

When I was 30, I averaged 70kg. After joining my company, I gained weight rapidly, and got up to 90kg, but when I was a freshman in my university, I weighed only 60kg.

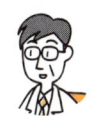

25 ドクター田中

糖尿病と診断するためには、ブドウ糖負荷試験を受けていただく必要があります。検査を受ける日に食べないで来てください。今日帰るときに、受付で検査日を予約してください。

I think it's necessary to check for diabetes mellitus, so you'll need to take a glucose tolerance test. Please don't have anything to eat the day you take the test. Could you make an appointment with the receptionist as you're leaving (when you leave) today?

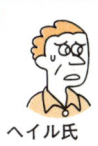

26 ヘイル氏

承知しました。

Certainly.

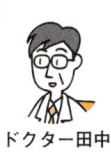

27 ドクター田中

私の知っている眼科の先生をご紹介しますので、次回の診察までに、そこで眼底検査を受けておいてください。

I'll refer you to an eye doctor I know, so you can take the eye ground test by the time you come back here.

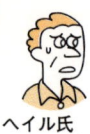

| 28 | ヘイル氏 | はい。
Yes, that sounds fine. |

| 29 | ドクター田中 | その時に心電図、肝機能、トリグリセライド、HDLコレステロールなども一緒に検査します。
Then, you'll take an electrocardiogram, along with a liver function test, and we'll measure your triglyceride and HDL cholesterol counts. |

| 30 | ヘイル氏 | わかりました。
I understand. |

| 31 | ドクター田中 | ブドウ糖負荷試験の結果が出る頃に、もう一度来院してください。それで、次にどうするかご相談しましょう。
① **When the result of the glucose tolerance test is available, please come here once more so we can discuss our next course of action.**
② **As soon as we know the result of the glucose tolerance test, I think you should come here again so we can discuss it.** |

| 32 | ヘイル氏 | ありがとうございました、先生。
Thank you very much, Doctor. |

| 33 | ドクター田中 | どういたしまして、お大事に。
Don't mention it. Take care of yourself. |

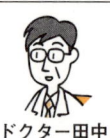

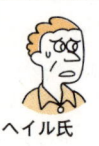

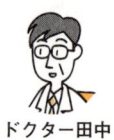

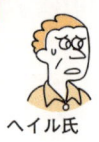

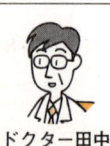

ちょっと一言 Medi Talk まとめ

Chapter 3 内科での英会話

皆さんが、患者さんを前にしてどんな会話が必要になるかを簡単な文章で考えてみましょう。口に出して発音してください。

待合室で待っている患者さんに対して

●お名前をお呼びするまで、椅子にかけてお待ちください。
　Please have a seat and wait until we call your name.

●気分はいかがですか？
　How do you feel now?

●今日は気分がよさそうですね。
　You look better today.

●わかりました。ちょっとお待ちください。
　Sure. Just a moment, please.

患者さんをフォローする際のやり取り

●この椅子にお座りください。
　Please take this seat.

●服を脱いで、このガウンに着替えてください。
　Please take off your clothes and put on this gown.

ちょっと一言 Medi Talk

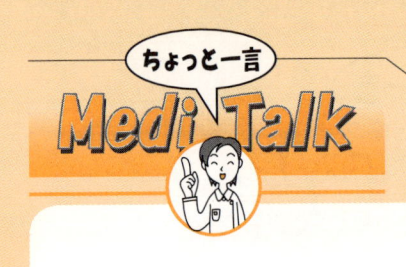

- 横になってください。
 Lie down, please.

- 立ってください。
 Stand up, please.

- 気分はよくなりましたか？
 Do you feel better?

- 全てうまくいっています。
 Everything is OK.

- うまくいくでしょう。
 Everything will be OK.

- ご心配なく。
 Don't worry.

- 落ち着いて。
 Calm down, please.

- 血液検査をします。
 You need a blood test.

- 袖をまくってください。
 Roll up your sleeve.

ちょっと一言 Medi Talk

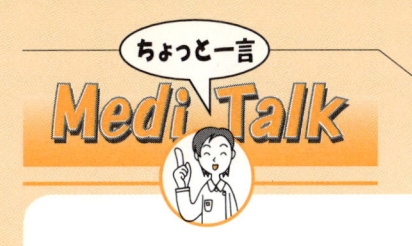

Chapter 3 内科での英会話

● 拳をしっかり握ってください。
Make a tight fist.

● ここを5分間ほど押さえていてください。
Press here for about 5 minutes.

● この容器に尿を入れてください。
Please urinate in this container.

● 終わったら、そこのコーナーに置いてください。
When you finish, put it in that corner.

診察後の患者さんに対して

● お大事に。
Take care of yourself.

● 刺激物はとらない方がいいでしょう。
You had better not have spicy food.

● よくならないようなら、再受診してください。
Come back if you don't feel better.

● 受付で次回の予約をしてください。
Make an appointment for the next time at the receptionist counter.

ちょっと一言 Medi Talk

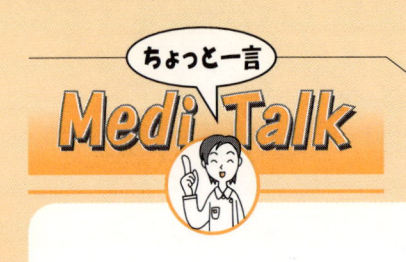

● 6月10日水曜日においでください。

Please come on Wednesday the 10th of June.

（書く場合は Wednesday 10th June となります）

● お薬 ＿＿＿ 日分の処方箋をお渡しします。

I'll give you a prescription for ＿＿＿ days.

● お薬の飲み方はわかりましたか？

Did you understand the directions about your medication?

● この薬でうがいをしてください。

Gargle with this medicine for the pain.

● きちんとお薬を飲まないとよくなりませんよ。

Take the medicine regularly, or you will not get better.

● タバコをやめませんか？ お力になれると思います。

Don't you want to quit smoking? We'll take care of you.

Chapter 4 CARDIOLOGY

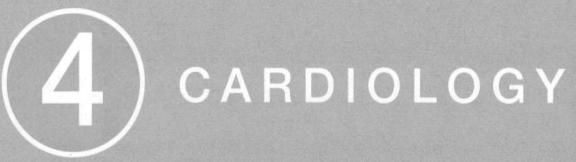

循環器科での英会話

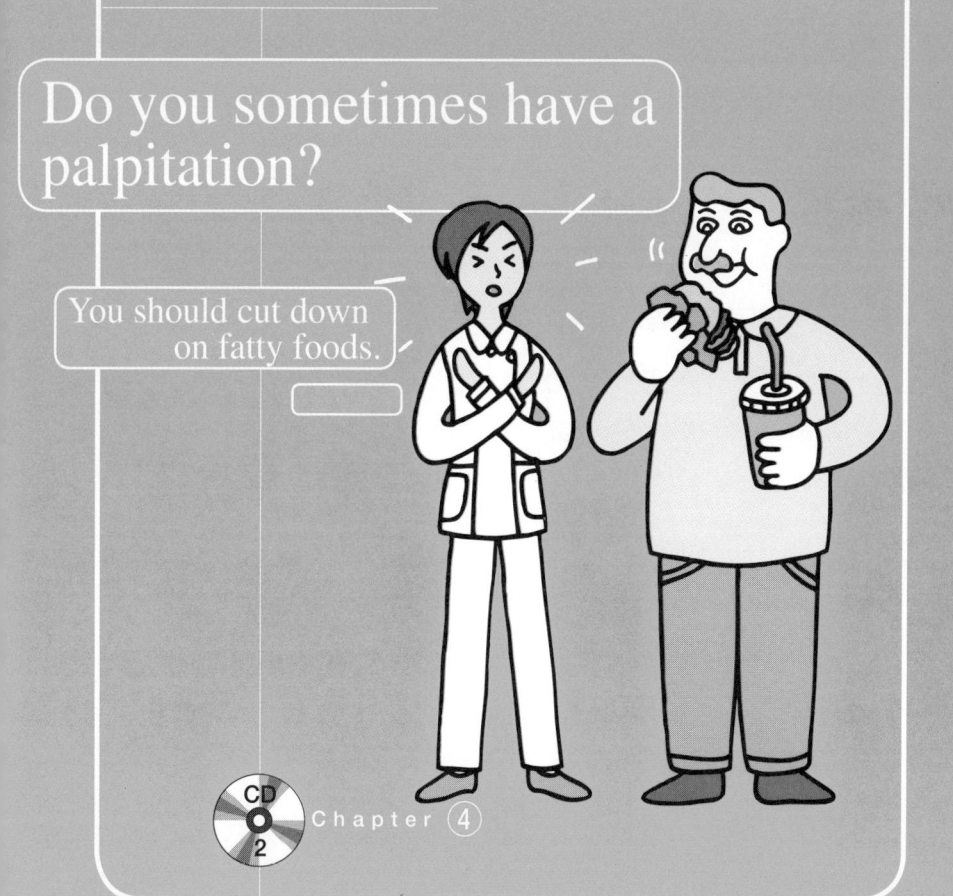

Do you sometimes have a palpitation?

You should cut down on fatty foods.

CD 2 Chapter 4

Chapter 4
CARDIOLOGY
循環器科での英会話

高血圧などの生活習慣病がますます増えています

先進国はどこの国でも、高血圧に代表される生活習慣病が大きな社会医学的な問題になっています。

日本でも過去数十年の間に、疾病構造が大きく変わり、特に高血圧は40年前に比べると、その発症率は3倍にもなっています。

それは、生活習慣の変化に伴い、社会的なストレスが大きくなったこと、運動不足や脂肪分・動物性蛋白のとりすぎ、食塩のとりすぎや、ファーストフードによる栄養の偏りが高血圧をますます増やしていると考えられています。

循環器疾患の患者さんに、どういった質問をしていくのか、考えてみましょう。

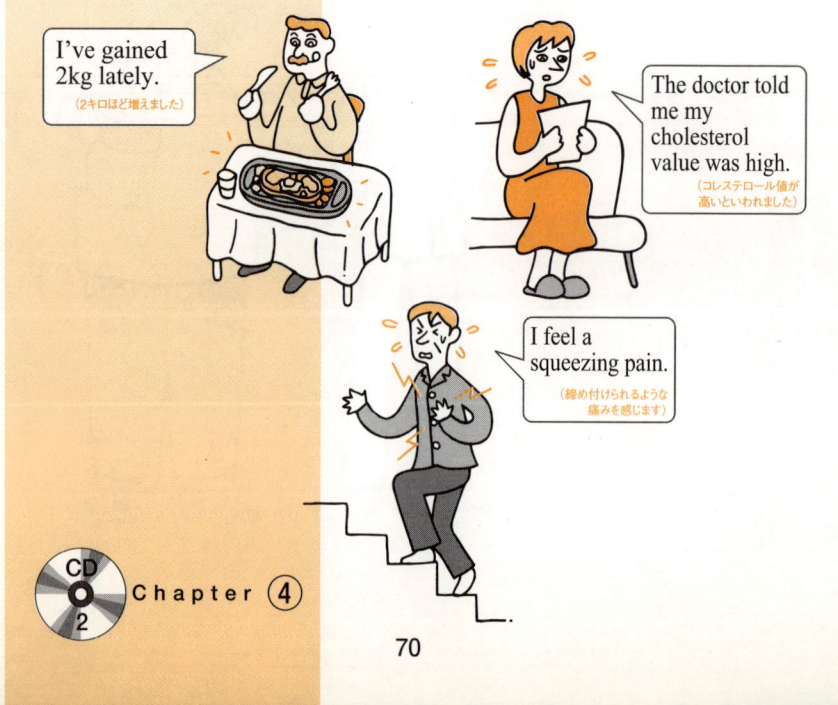

I've gained 2kg lately.
（2キロほど増えました）

The doctor told me my cholesterol value was high.
（コレステロール値が高いといわれました）

I feel a squeezing pain.
（締め付けられるような痛みを感じます）

ちょっと一言 Medi Talk

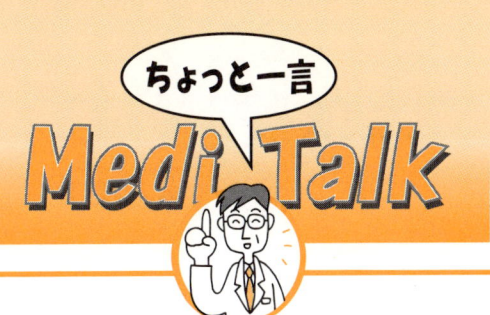

●何か症状はありますか？
Do you have any symptoms?

●めまいを起こしたことがありますか？
Have you ever had dizziness?

●動悸はしませんか？
Do you sometimes have a palpitation?

●息切れはしませんか？
Do you have shortness of breath?

●軽い運動はできますか？
Can you tolerate mild exercise?

●例えば、階段を息もつかないで昇れますか？
For instance, can you climb up a flight of stairs without pausing for breath?

●動悸がしたり、脈が速くなったりすることがありますか？
Do you sometimes have a palpitation or a fast heart beat?

●体重に変化はありませんか？
Have you noticed any change of your body weight?

ちょっと一言 Medi Talk

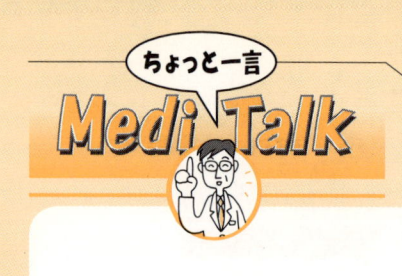

●下肢や下腹部にむくみが出たことがありますか？
Have you noticed any swelling in your legs or lower abdomen?

●医師から心臓病があると言われたことがありますか？
Has it ever been pointed out that you had a heart disease?

●あなたの主治医から心臓が悪いと言われたことがありますか？
Have you ever been told by your doctor that you had a heart disease?

●心臓に雑音があると言われたことがありますか？
Has it ever been pointed out to you that you had a heart murmur?

●あなたの血圧はいかがですか？ 正常ですか、それとも正常より少し高めですか？
How is your blood pressure? Is it normal, or a little higher than normal?

●脈拍と血圧を測ります。
I'm going to take your pulse and blood pressure.

●あなたの血圧は、125/85mmHgです。
Your blood pressure is 125/85mmHg.

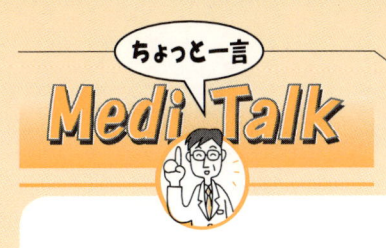

● 今までに血圧が高いと言われたことはありますか？
Have you ever been told before that your blood pressure was high?

● ご両親は高血圧になったことがありますか？
Do your parents have a history of high blood pressure?

● ご両親やご兄弟（姉妹）で心臓の悪い方はいらっしゃいますか？
Do you have any family members who have heart trouble?

● 何かお薬を服用なさっていますか？
Do you take any medicines now?

● 以前に胸痛がありましたか？
Have you ever had any chest pain?

● 胸の痛みは今までに比べ、軽いですか、同じくらいですか、もっと強い痛みですか？
Compared with the previous chest pain, is this mild, the same or more severe?

● どこが痛いですか？　痛いところを指差してください。
Where is your pain? Point to where it hurts.

Medi Talk　ちょっと一言

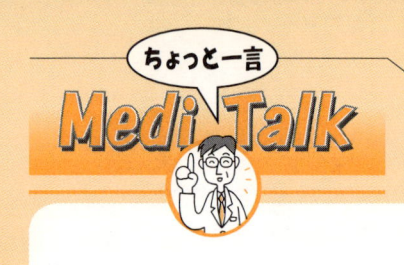

●痛みは肩やあごの方に広がりましたか？

Did the pain travel to your shoulder or jaw?

●医師から処方された薬を飲んでいますか？

Do you take medicine prescribed by a doctor?

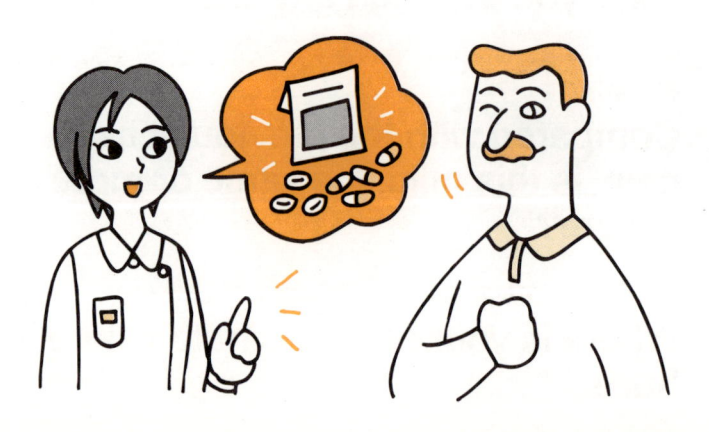

MediTalk

高血圧
High blood pressure (Hypertension)

Chapter 4 循環器科での英会話

ケリーさんが、健康診断で血圧が高いと指摘されたため、田中クリニックを訪れました。

Mr. Kelly visited the Tanaka Clinic, because he found out he had high blood pressure from a routine physical check up.

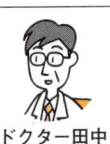

---

1 ドクター田中

どうされました?

① What seems to be the trouble?

② How can I help you today?

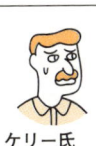

---

2 ケリー氏

先日健康診断を受けた時、少し血圧が高いので、一度診てもらった方がいいと言われました。

① When I had a physical examination recently, the doctor said that my blood pressure was a little high and that I should see another doctor.

② My blood pressure was slightly high in my last check up, and I was advised to see another doctor.

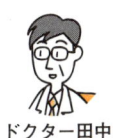

---

3 ドクター田中

それはいつのことですか?

① When was it checked?

② When was that?

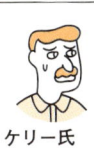

---

4 ケリー氏

2週間くらい前です。

About two weeks ago.

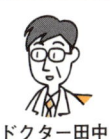

---

5 ドクター田中

何か症状はありますか?

① Do you have any symptoms?

② Any special symptoms?

6 ケリー氏

特にありません。

① Nothing special.

② Nothing in particular.

③ Nothing comes to mind.

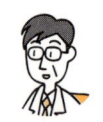

---

7 ドクター田中

今まで血圧が高いと言われたことはありますか？ あるいは降圧剤を飲んだことがありますか？

Were you ever told before that your blood pressure was high? Or have you ever taken depressants before?

---

8 ケリー氏

何度か少し高いと言われたことはありますが、降圧剤を飲んだことはありません。

Some doctors said that my blood pressure was a little high, but I haven't taken any depressants.

---

9 ドクター田中

何かほかの病気にかかったことがありますか？

Have you had any other illnesses?

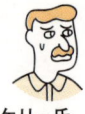

---

10 ケリー氏

特に重い病気にかかったことはありません。

I have never had anything serious, Doctor.

---

11 ドクター田中

あなたのご両親は高血圧の既往歴がありますか？ あるいは近親者で脳卒中や心筋梗塞を起こした方はいませんか？

Has there been an incidence of high blood pressure in your parents, or have any relatives suffered from a stroke or a heart attack?

12 ケリー氏

実は、私の父は昨年心筋梗塞で亡くなりました。

① **To be honest with you, my father died of a heart attack last year.**

② **To tell the truth, my father passed away after a heart attack last year.**

13 ドクター田中

それはお気の毒に。ところで生活は規則正しい方ですか？ タバコやお酒はどうですか？

① **That's too bad.**

② **I'm sorry to hear that.**

By the way, would you say that you live a normal lifestyle? And what about smoking or drinking?

14 ケリー氏

責任の重い仕事についているせいか、時々眠れないことがあり、寝る前にしばしばお酒を飲みます。しかし、タバコの方は2年前にやめました。

Sometimes I suffer from insomnia because of the responsibilities of my job, so I often have a drink before bed. However, I quit smoking two years ago.

15 ドクター田中

最近、体重が減ったり増えたりということはありませんか？

① **Have you lost or gained weight recently?**

② **Has your weight changed recently?**

16 ケリー氏

2キロほど増えました。

① **I noticed that I've gained 2kg lately.**

② **I seem to have put on 2kg lately.**

17 ドクター田中

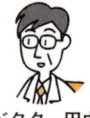

わかりました。ちょっと診察してみましょう。楽にしてください。

① I see. Well, I'd like to examine you. Just relax.

② I see. Well, let's have a look at you. Just relax.

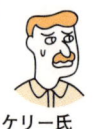

18 ケリー氏

はい、先生。

Okay, Doctor.

19 ドクター田中

（診察をした後、ドクター田中はケリー氏に向かって）
健康診断で指摘されたように、あなたの血圧は正常よりやや高めですね。いくつかの検査をしてみましょう。検査室の方へどうぞ。

As the other doctor indicated, your blood pressure is a little above normal. I'd like to run some tests. Please go into that lab. to be tested.

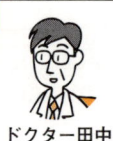

20 ドクター田中

（検査が終わって、ケリー氏はもう一度、ドクター田中に面談します）
本態性の高血圧かもしれません。

① You seem to have essential hypertension.

② It looks like you may have essential hypertension.

21 ドクター田中

1週間後に検査結果をお知らせします。その時まで塩分の多い食事は避け、お酒も飲みすぎないようにしてください。何か質問はありませんか？

I'll tell you the results of the tests in a week. Until I see you here again, you should cut down on salty foods and drinking. Do you have any questions?

Chapter 4 循環器科での英会話

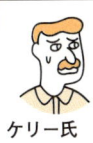

22 ケリー氏

高血圧は危険な病気なのでしょうか？

① **Is high blood pressure a serious condition?**

② **Is high blood pressure dangerous?**

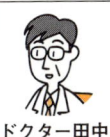

23 ドクター田中

ご心配でしょうが、そんなに気にする必要はありません。容易に治療できますし、コントロールも容易です。

It's a cause for concern, but don't worry too much about it. It can be treated easily and kept under control.

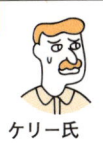

24 ケリー氏

それを聞いて安心しました。どうもありがとうございました。

① **I'm relieved to hear that. Thank you, Doctor.**

② **I'm so happy to hear that. Thank you, Doctor.**

③ **What a relief！ Thank you, Doctor.**

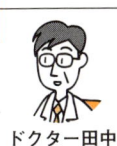

25 ドクター田中

お大事に。また来週お会いしましょう。

Take it easy. See you next week.

MediTalk

狭心症
Angina pectoris

バーガーさんが、1か月前から胸痛が起こるようになり、田中クリニックを訪れました。

Mr. Burger visited the Tanaka Clinic, because of a gradual onset of chest pain lasting for a month.

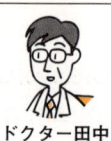

---

1 ドクター田中

今日はどうなさったのですか?

What can I do for you today?

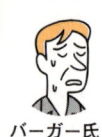

---

2 バーガー氏

急に階段を駆け上がったりすると胸の中心部に締め付けられるような痛みを感じます。

① **I feel a squeezing pain in the center of my chest when I run up stairs rapidly.**

② **I feel a tightness in my chest when I climb stairs quickly.**

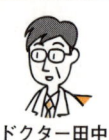

---

3 ドクター田中

いつ頃から感じ始めましたか? いつもどのぐらい続きますか?

① **When did you first feel it? How long does it continue usually?**

② **When did it begin? How long does the pain usually last?**

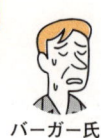

---

4 バーガー氏

1か月ぐらい前に最初に感じました。いつも2分間ぐらい続きます。

① **I first felt it about a month ago. It usually hurts for a couple of minutes.**

② **I noticed it for the first time around a month ago. The pain usually lasts for a couple of minutes.**

Chapter 4 循環器科での英会話

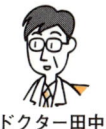

5 ドクター田中
以前より痛みの頻度は増えていませんか？ あるいは痛みの度合いは以前より悪くなっていませんか？

① Have you been feeling it more often lately, or has the pain become worse than before?

② Has the frequency of the pain increased recently, or has it become more intense than it was at first?

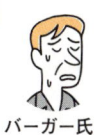

6 バーガー氏
特に変化はありません。

① It hasn't changed particularly.

② I haven't noticed any changes, really.

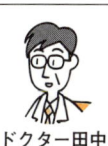

7 ドクター田中
以前、何かほかの病気にかかったことがありますか？

① Have you had any other illnesses before?

② Have you had any other health problems in the past?

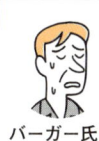

8 バーガー氏
いいえ。ただ健康診断のとき、血圧が高いと言われました。

① No, I haven't, although I was told I have high blood pressure in my last physical examination.

② No, never, but I found out in my last check up that my blood pressure was high.

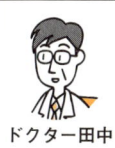

9 ドクター田中
ご家族はいかがですか？ 心臓病の方はいませんか？

① How is your family medical history? Has anyone suffered from a heart disease?

81

② Can you tell me about your family medical history? Has there been any incidence of a heart disease?

---

10 バーガー氏

父が心筋梗塞のため昨年、入院しました。

① My father was hospitalized for a heart attack last year.

② My father had a heart attack last year.

---

11 ドクター田中

それはいけませんね。ところで、お酒やタバコはいかがですか?

I'm sorry to hear that. By the way, do you drink or smoke?

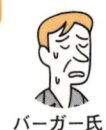

---

12 バーガー氏

会社のつきあいなどのほかは、そうたびたび飲みません。しかし、タバコはストレスが多いせいか、1日2箱以上吸います。

① I don't drink very often except at business gatherings, but I smoke over 2 packs of cigarettes a day, because my job is very stressful.

② I only drink with my coworkers or business clients, but I smoke over 2 packs of cigarettes a day, because my job is very stressful.

---

13 ドクター田中

ちょっと吸いすぎのようですね。とにかく診てみましょう。シャツを脱いでいただけますか?

I think you smoke too much. Anyway, let's have a look at you. Would you mind removing your shirt?

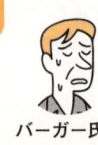

---

14 バーガー氏

はい、先生。

Okay, Doctor.

Chapter 4 循環器科での英会話

15 ドクター田中
(ドクター田中はバーガー氏を診察した後、検査を行うことにしました)
心電図であなたの心臓を調べてみましょう。

I'd like to take an electrocardiogram now to check your heart.

16 ドクター田中
(心電図をとった後、それをチェックしながら)
安静時の心電図に問題はありません。それでは次に、運動した後、あなたの脈拍数がどうなるか診てみましょう。

Your heart looks all right when you're at rest and relaxed. Let's take another one after you exert a little to elevate your heart beat.

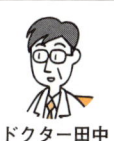

17 ドクター田中
(運動負荷テストの後)
何か胸に痛みを感じましたか？

① **Did you feel any pain in your chest?**

② **Any discomfort in your chest?**

18 バーガー氏
はい、締め付けられるような痛みを感じました。ただ、それはいつもより軽いものでしたが。

① **Yes, I felt a squeezing pain, but it was lighter than usual.**

② **Yes, I felt the same squeezing pain, but it wasn't as strong as usual.**

19 ドクター田中
(心電図を見ながら)
心電図検査の結果によると、あなたは労作性狭心症のようです。

According to the result of this electrocardiogram, you seem to have angina pectoris during exertion.

20 バーガー氏

それはどんな病気ですか？ 重い病気なのでしょうか？

What is it? Is it a serious condition?

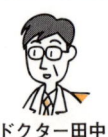

---

21 ドクター田中

心臓を取り巻く血管の動脈硬化によって起こる病気です。しかし、薬で容易にコントロールできます。

It's due to hardening of the arteries surrounding the heart. It can be controlled easily though, with medication.

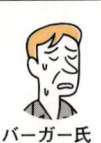

---

22 バーガー氏

心臓の弁の病気ではないのですね？

It is not a leaky valve, is it?

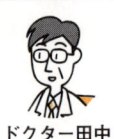

---

23 ドクター田中

そうです。ただし、なるべく早く専門病院で精密検査を受け、治療方針を決定した方がよいでしょう。

That's right. It isn't. However, you should have a more detailed examination taken as soon as possible by a cardiologist who can decide on an effective course of treatment.

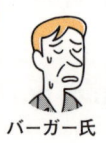

---

24 バーガー氏

わかりました。ところで日常生活ではどんなことに気をつけたらよいでしょうか？

① **I see, Doctor. Well, what changes should I make in my daily life?**

② **All right, Doctor. Will I need to make any changes in my daily life?**

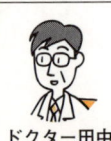

---

25 ドクター田中

できるだけ早くタバコをやめるようにしてください。そして、脂肪分の多い食べ物も減らしてください。

You should quit smoking as soon as possible, and cut down on fatty foods.

| 26 | バーガー氏 | わかりました。
I understand. |

| 27 | ドクター田中 | 2種類の薬を出しましょう。この薬を1日2回2錠ずつ、それからこの薬は発作が起きたときに1錠飲んでください。
I'll give you two types of tablets. Take two of these twice a day and take one of the other tablets if an attack happens. |

| 28 | バーガー氏 | わかりました、先生。
Okay, Doctor. |

| 29 | ドクター田中 | それから、心臓病の専門医をしている私の友人がいる病院がありますから、紹介してあげましょう。
I'll refer you to my friend at a hospital who is a specialist in heart disease. |

| 30 | バーガー氏 | どうもありがとうございました。
① **Thank you very much, Doctor.**
② **I can't thank you enough, Doctor.** |

| 31 | ドクター田中 | どういたしまして。お大事に。
Don't mention it. Take care of yourself. |

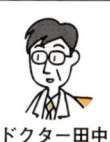

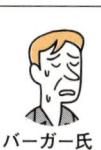

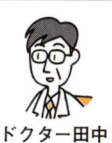

MediTalk

高脂血症
Hyper-lipidemia

アンダーソンさんが、健康診断の結果、コレステロール値が高いと指摘されたため、田中クリニックを訪れました。

Ms. Anderson visited the Tanaka Clinic, because it was pointed out that she had high cholesterol in a routine physical check up.

1 ドクター田中

どうなさいました?
What can I do for you today?

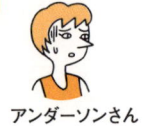

2 アンダーソンさん

先日、健康診断でコレステロール値が高いと言われました。

① **When I had a physical examination recently, the doctor said my cholesterol was high.**

② **The doctor who examined me recently in a physical check up told me my cholesterol value was high.**

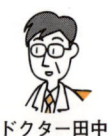

3 ドクター田中

どのくらい高かったですか?
How high was it?

4 アンダーソンさん

280mg/dlあると言われました。
It was 280mg/dl.

5 ドクター田中

トリグリセライドやHDLは測りましたか?
Did he examine your triglyceride or HDL cholesterol?

6 アンダーソンさん

いいえ、測りませんでした。
No, he didn't.

7 ドクター田中

ほかにどんな検査を受けましたか？

① Did he check anything else?

② What else did he look at?

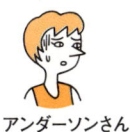

8 アンダーソンさん

血圧とか肝機能です。

① Yes, he examined my blood pressure and liver function.

② He checked my blood pressure as well as my liver function.

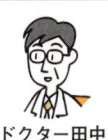

9 ドクター田中

それらに、何か異常はありましたか？

How were the results?

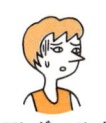

10 アンダーソンさん

特にありませんでした。

① Nothing special.

② There didn't seem to be anything wrong.

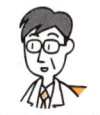

11 ドクター田中

ご家族の中で心臓病の方はいらっしゃいますか？

① Have any family members suffered from a heart disease?

② Has there been any incidence of heart disease in your family?

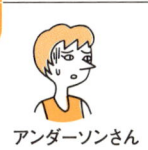

12 アンダーソンさん

実は数年前、父が心筋梗塞で亡くなりました。

① To be honest with you, my father passed away from a heart attack a few years ago.

② I'm almost afraid to say it, but my father died of a heart attack a few years ago.

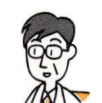

---

13 ドクター田中

それはお気の毒に。おいくつで亡くなられたのですか？

① That's too bad. How old was he?

② I'm sorry to hear that. How old was he?

---

14 アンダーソンさん

64歳でした。

① He was 64 years old.

② At the time he was 64.

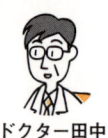

---

15 ドクター田中

ところで、今まで何か大きな病気をしたことがありますか？

By the way, have you ever had any other serious illnesses?

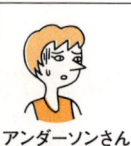

---

16 アンダーソンさん

特にありません。

Never anything serious, Doctor.

---

17 ドクター田中

自覚症状はありますか？　例えば胸が痛かったりとか、脚が痛かったりとか？

① Do you have any symptoms? For instance, chest pain or leg pain?

② For instance, have you experienced pain in your chest or legs recently?

Chapter 4

循環器科での英会話

18 アンダーソンさん

特にありません。
① No, I haven't.
② No, not that I can remember.

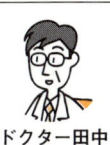

19 ドクター田中

お酒やタバコはいかがですか?
Do you smoke or drink?

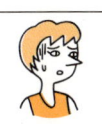

20 アンダーソンさん

タバコは1箱ぐらい、お酒は1日ビール1本ぐらいです。
① Yes, I usually smoke around 1 pack of cigarettes and drink 1 bottle of beer a day.
② I hate to say it, but yes. A pack of cigarettes and a bottle of beer a day.

21 ドクター田中

それでは、ちょっと診察してみましょう。シャツを脱いでいただけますか?
① Anyway, I'd like to examine you. Would you mind taking your shirt off, please?
② I see. Well, let's have a look at you. Would you mind removing your shirt, please?

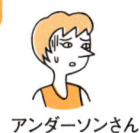

22 アンダーソンさん

はい。
No, not at all.

23 ドクター田中

(診察した後)
次に眼底を診ますので、ちょっと部屋を暗くします。
Next, I'd like to see your eye ground. Let me turn off the light.

24 ドクター田中

コレステロールやHDLのもっと詳しい検査をするため、これから採血します。右の袖をまくっていただけますか？

① I'd like to do a blood test now to get a more detailed breakdown of your cholesterol and HDL cholesterol counts. Could you roll up your right sleeve?

② Now I'd like to take a little blood in order to get a more accurate, detailed value of your cholesterol and HDL cholesterol levels. Roll up your right sleeve, please.

25 ドクター田中

（検査の後）
1週間後の同じ時間にもう一度来院してください。結果をお知らせします。

Please come back in a week at the same time. I'll tell you the results of the tests then.

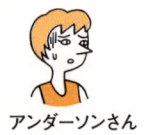

26 アンダーソンさん

わかりました。ところでこの1週間、どう過ごしたらいいでしょうか？

① Okay, Doctor. Do I need to make any changes in my daily life between now and then?

② That sounds good, Doctor. Do I have to do anything special until then regarding my daily routine?

27 ドクター田中

今診たところ、コレステロール以外には異常はないようです。

According to the examination I did, you don't seem to have anything wrong with you except a high cholesterol value.

28 アンダーソンさん

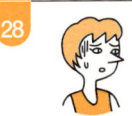

それを聞いて何よりです。
I am glad to hear that.

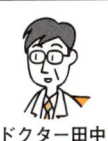

29 ドクター田中

次回は、食事療法などこれからの対策をお話しします。それまでは今までどおりの生活で結構です。
I'll advise you about recommended foods and so on next time, so you may lead a normal life until then.

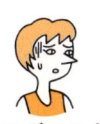

30 アンダーソンさん

どうもありがとうございました、先生。
Thank you very much, Doctor.

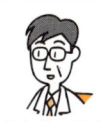

31 ドクター田中

どういたしまして。どうかあまり気になさらないように。
You're welcome. Please don't worry too much about it.

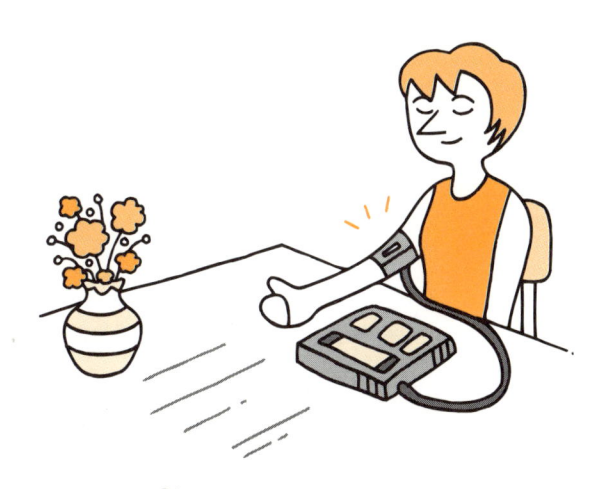

内科・循環器科用語

あ

アイゼンメンジャー症候群	Eisenmenger's complex
アシドーシス	acidosis
アナフィラキシー（過敏症）	anaphylaxis
アミロイド腫	amyloid tumor
アルカローシス	alkalosis
一次孔	ostium primum
溢血	extravasation
うずくまる	squat
うなるような	roaring
運動失調症	ataxia
会陰	perineum
壊死	necrosis
エストロゲン	estrogen
円錐部	conus
円柱腫	cylindroma
遅い	slow

か

解離	lysis
拡張期	diastolic period
下行大動脈	descending aorta
過伸展	hyperextension
滑液濃縮	synovial thickening
癌	carcinoma
間欠性無収縮	intermittent asystole
間欠熱	intermittent fever
感受性	susceptibility
関節症	arthropathy
肝脾腫	hepatosplenomegaly
陥没臓器	hollow viscus
奇異な行動	eccentricities of manner
気管	trachea
気管支鏡	bronchoscopy
奇形	malformation
偽囊胞	pseudocyst
脚ブロック	bundle branch block

逆行性	retrograde
吸引する	aspirate
仰臥位	supine position
胸郭	thorax
胸骨縁	sternal border
棘球虫（包虫）	Echinococcus
近接様効果（EKG上）	intrinsicoid deflection
空洞の、くぼんだ	hollow
軀幹	trunk
形成不全	hypoplasia
頸動脈	carotid artery
血圧	blood pressure
血圧計	sphygmomanometer
血液側路	blood shunt
血管陰影	vascular shadow
血管輪	vascular ring
血行動態	hemodynamics
結紮	ligation
結節性紅斑	erythema nodosum
血栓性静脈炎	thrombophlebitis
結滞	pulse deficit
結膜	conjunctiva
検体	specimen
高血圧	high blood pressure, hypertension
好酸球増多症	eosinophilia
甲状腺機能亢進症	hyperthyroidism
甲状腺中毒症	thyrotoxicosis
後前位の	posteroanterior (PA)
酵素	enzyme
呼吸困難	dyspnea
姑息的	palliative
骨盤の入り口	pelvic brim

さ

最高血圧	maximum blood pressure
最低血圧	minimum blood pressure

鎖骨	clavicle
鎖骨下動脈	subclavian artery
三尖弁閉鎖	tricuspid atresia
持続熱	continuous fever
弛張熱	remittent fever
失神	syncope
脂肪腫	lipoma
死亡率	mortality rate
充血	hyperemia
収縮期	systolic period
収縮期雑音	systolic murmur
収縮期スリル	systolic thrill
縮窄	constriction
障害、中断	interruption
障害された	handicapped
上行大動脈	ascending aorta
衝突	collision
静脈波図	venogram
食道	esophagus
食道後部大動脈	retroesophageal aorta
人工心肺	cardiopulmonary bypass
心雑音	heart murmur
心耳	auricle
心室中隔欠損	ventricular septal defect (VSD)
心室吻合術	ventriculostomy
滲出液	effusion
新生物（腫瘍）	neoplasm
心臓カテーテル	cardiac catheterization
心臓血管撮影	angiocardiography
心臓停止	cardiac standstill
心臓弁尖	valve cusp
心電図	electrocardiogram
心内膜炎	endocarditis
心房中隔欠損	atrial septal defect (ASD)
じんま疹	urticaria
心理的な	psychogenic

膵臓炎	pancreatitis
水平面	horizontal plane
整	regular
生検	biopsy
正常	normal
正常以下	subnormal
切開する	incise
赤血球増加症	polycythemia
赤血球沈降速度	blood sedimentation rate
セミ・ファウラー体位	semi-Fowler's position
前胸部	precordium
先天性心臓血管奇形	congenital cardiovascular anomalies
喘鳴	stridor
造影剤	radiopaque fluid
側胸骨部	parasternal area
側副循環	collateral circulation
そ径上部	suprainguinal region
組織学	histology
そ嚢	crop

た

体型	habitus
大腿骨	femur
大腿動脈飽和	femoral arterial saturation
大動脈弓	aortic arch
大動脈撮影	aortography
大動脈縮窄	coarctation of aorta
大動脈転位	transposition of great vessels
大動脈弁狭窄	aortic stenosis
多血球症	polycythemia
棚様突出	shelf-like protrusion
多発関節炎	polyarthritis
断層撮影	tomography
チアノーゼの	cyanotic
窒息	choking

中断、障害	interruption
徴候	episode
腸骨動脈	iliac artery
聴診	auscultation
強い	strong, intense, hard
低血圧	low blood pressure, hypotension
低体温	hypothermia
定量の	quantitative
転移	metastases
動悸	palpitation
透視検査法	fluoroscopy
動脈管開存症	patent ductus arteriosus
動脈瘤	aneurysm
特発性	idiopathic
時計軸回転	clockwise rotation
凸（とつ）	convexity

な

内臓破裂	visceral rupture
二次孔開存	persistent ostium secondum
乳酸脱水素酵素	lactic dehydrogenase
嚢腫	cyst

は

肺断層撮影	lung scan
肺動脈輪	pulmonary annulus
肺門部血管	hilar vessels
拍動性の	pulsatile
ばち状指	clubbed finger
速い	rapid, fast
バリウム	barium
半坐位	half sitting
比重	specific gravity
肥大	hypertrophy
肥満	obese

病理解剖	autopsy
び爛（ただれ）	erosion
頻脈	tachycardia
ファロー四徴症	tetralogy of Fallot
腹臥位	lying on stomach
腹膜炎	peritonitis
浮腫	edema
不整	irregular
普通	ordinal
吻合	anastomosis
分離	crisis
分裂	division
閉鎖	atresia
閉塞	occlusion
ベクトル心電図	vectorcardiogram
ヘマトクリット	hematocrit
ヘモグロビン	hemoglobin
扁平足	flat foot
弁膜切開	valvulotomy
弁膜の狭窄	valvular stenosis
剖検	necropsy
包虫	Echinococcus
歩行	gait
発作性呼吸困難	paroxysmal dyspnea

ま

末端浮腫	peripheral edema
脈	pulse
脈圧	pulse pressure
脈波	pulse wave
脈拍数	pulse rate
無害性雑音/機能性雑音	innocent murmur/functional murmur
無呼吸	apnea
無症状の	asymptomatic
無名動脈	innominate artery

メトヘモグロビン血症	methemoglobinemia

や

やせ型	sthenia
癒着交連	fused commissures
予防的	prophylactic
弱い	weak, feeble, thready

ら

卵円孔開存	patent foramen ovale
リパーゼ	lipase
類肉腫	sarcoid
レントゲン写真	roentgenogram
漏斗状の	infundibular type
肋骨の切痕	notching of the ribs

わ

腕頭動脈	truncus brachiocephalicus

Chapter 5
SURGERY
ORTHOPEDICS

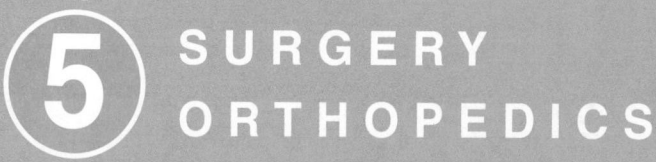

外科・整形外科での英会話

Where is your pain?

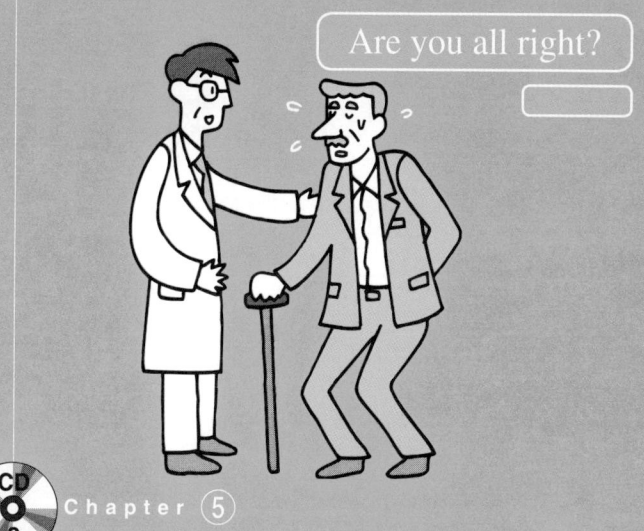

Are you all right?

Chapter 5

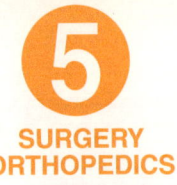

SURGERY ORTHOPEDICS

外科・整形外科での英会話

高齢の方が増え、腰痛はよく見られる症状です

　最近、高齢者の方が受診される率が高くなり、狭心症などの虚血性心疾患が日常的に見られるようになりました。同時に、加齢により腰や膝などの運動器にも障害を起こす率が高くなってきました。この章では、日常よく見られる腰痛を取り上げてみました。

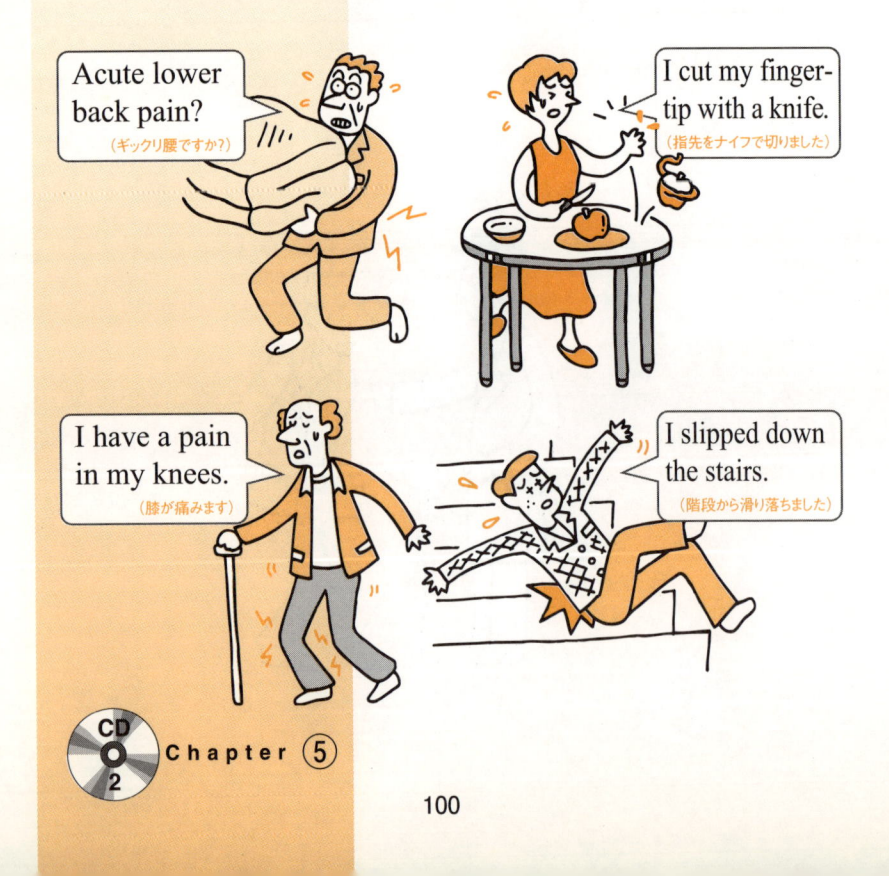

Acute lower back pain?
（ギックリ腰ですか?）

I cut my fingertip with a knife.
（指先をナイフで切りました）

I have a pain in my knees.
（膝が痛みます）

I slipped down the stairs.
（階段から滑り落ちました）

CD 2　Chapter ⑤

ちょっと一言 Medi Talk

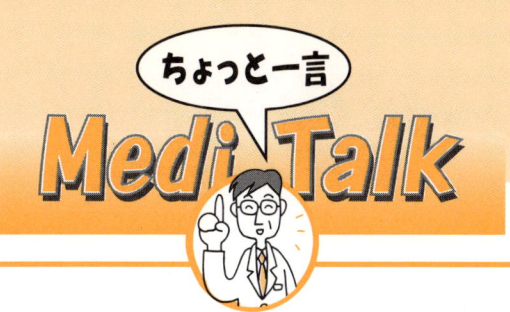

●いつ痛めましたか？
When did you hurt yourself?

●どこが痛いですか？　痛いところを指差してください。
Where is your pain?
Point to where it hurts.

●どこを打ちましたか？　打ったところを指差してください。
Where did you hit yourself?
Point to where you hit yourself.

●痛みますか？
Does it hurt?

●押さえると痛いですか？
Does it hurt when I press it?

●大丈夫ですか？
Are you all right?

●よく背中が痛みますか？
Do you have a backache frequently?

●歩き始めるときに、膝が痛みますか？
Do you have any pain in your knees when you start to walk?

Chapter 5
外科・整形外科での英会話

ちょっと一言 Medi Talk

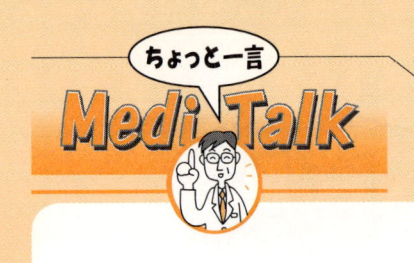

- 肩こりがありますか？
  Do you have shoulder stiffness?

- どのくらい痛みが続いていますか？
  How long have you had this pain?

- 大丈夫ですよ。
  You will be OK.

- 怪我をしたのですか？
  Does anything hurt?

- どこをけがしましたか？　見せてください。
  Where? Show me.

- 階段から滑り落ちました。
  I slipped down the stairs.

- 指先を料理ナイフで切りました。
  I cut my fingertip with a kitchen knife.

- 腕を骨折しました。
  I got a fracture of my arm.

- 昨日、右足首を捻挫しました。
  I sprained my right ankle yesterday.

Chapter 5 外科・整形外科での英会話

ちょっと一言 Medi Talk

● 傷口を清潔にしてください。
You must keep the wound clean.

● 傷の消毒をします。
I will clean up your wound.

● ガーゼを変えます。
I will change the gauze.

● 専門の先生を呼んできます。
I am calling a specialist to see you.

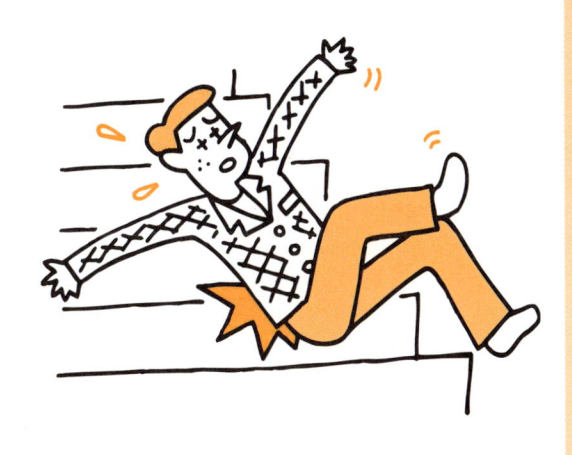

MediTalk

腰痛 / Lumbago

ジェームスさんが、田中クリニックにやって来ました。どうも腰が痛そうです。

Mr. James visited the Tanaka Clinic. He seems to have a lower backache.

---

1 ドクター田中

どうされましたか?

What seems to be the trouble?

---

2 ジェームス氏

昨日の朝起きようとしたら、急に腰に痛みを感じ、それ以来体を自由に動かせなくて1日中うちで横になっていました。

① **When I was getting out of bed yesterday morning, I suddenly felt a pain in my lower back. Since I wasn't able to move easily, I decided to stay home and rest all day long.**

② **I felt a pain in my lower back while trying to get up yesterday morning. It was so bad, I couldn't get out of bed all day.**

---

3 ドクター田中

痛みは昨日より今日の方がひどいですか?

① **Has the pain become more severe than it was yesterday?**

② **Is the pain worse now than it was?**

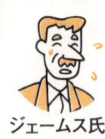

---

4 ジェームス氏

いいえ、次第にやわらいでいるようです。ベッドから起き上がれるようになりましたので、今日こうしてこのクリニックに足を引きずりながらでも来ることができました。

① **No, it seems to be decreasing gradually, so I was able to move well enough to get out of bed and drag myself to this clinic.**

② **It's not quite as bad as it was, so I was able to get up and come here.**

Chapter 5

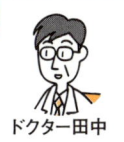

5 ドクター田中

いつ痛みが強くなりますか？ 休んでいる時ですか？ それとも起き上がる時ですか？

① When is the pain worse, while resting or when trying to get up?

② Is it more painful when you're at rest, or when you're trying to get up?

6 ジェームス氏

ほとんど同じくらいです。

① It's basically the same, no matter what I do.

② I don't think there's any difference.

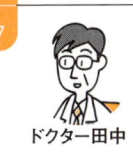

7 ドクター田中

ところで、その痛みはズキズキする痛みですか？ 鋭い痛みですか？ それとも鈍い痛みですか？

Would you describe the feeling as a throbbing pain, a sharp pain, or a dull pain?

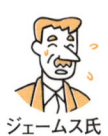

8 ジェームス氏

かなり鋭い痛みです。

It's quite a sharp pain.

9 ドクター田中

脚がしびれたり、痛みが脚の方に広がることはありませんか？

① Have you felt any numbness in your legs, or has the pain spread down into your legs?

② Have you felt any numbness or pain in your legs?

10 ジェームス氏

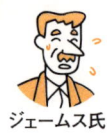

いいえ、ありません。

① No, I haven't felt anything wrong in my legs.

② No, I haven't felt anything strange in my legs.

11 ドクター田中

それでは診察してみましょう。シャツとズボンを脱いでください。そして、後ろ向きに立ってください。

Okay. I'd like to examine you now, so would you please take off your shirt and trousers and stand with your back towards me?

12 ジェームス氏

はい、先生。

All right, Doctor.

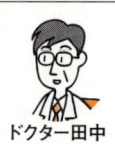

13 ドクター田中

（診察した後）
あなたの痛みは筋肉性の腰痛が原因のようです。しかし念のため、レントゲンを撮ってみましょう。

① I think you're suffering from muscular lower back pain, but we'll take an X-ray to be sure.

② It looks to me like a case of muscular lower back pain, but to verify that we'll need to take an X-ray.

14 ジェームス氏

はい、先生。

Okay, Doctor.

15 ドクター田中

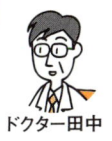

（レントゲン検査を済ませた後）
レントゲンの結果では、やはり変形性脊椎症や椎間板ヘルニアのような骨、関節の疾患ではないようです。

This X-ray doesn't indicate any evidence of a bone or joint related disease, like spondylosis deformans or intervertebral disc hernia.

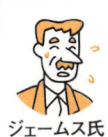

16 ジェームス氏

そうですか。では、なぜ痛むのですか？

Is that right?
Then, why have I got a pain in my back?

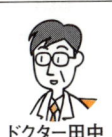

17 ドクター田中

つまり、レントゲン上には何の異常も見られません。筋肉性の急性の腰痛、いわゆるギックリ腰のようです。

In other words, there's nothing abnormal about your X-ray. It looks like the pain's coming from the muscles in your lower back. The condition is known as "acute lower back pain".

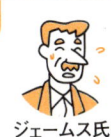

18 ジェームス氏

ギックリ腰ですか？

Acute lower back pain?

19 ドクター田中

そうです。それでは、この筋肉の痛みと緊張を取る薬を1日3回服用し、また、この湿布薬を1日2回腰に貼ってください。

That's right. I'm going to prescribe these analgesics (pain killer) and muscle relaxants which I want you to take three times a day, and apply this warm compress twice a day to your lower back.

20 ジェームス氏

薬を1日に3回も飲むのですか?
Do I have to take the drug 3 times a day?

21 ドクター田中

そうです。腰に弾性包帯を巻けば動きやすいでしょう。腰を保護しておけば仕事をしてもよいでしょう。

① **That's right. It'll be easier for you to move if you wrap your lower back with an elastic support bandage. That will allow you to go back to work right away.**

② **I recommend that you wear an elastic support bandage around your waist so you can move easier and go back to work soon.**

22 ジェームス氏

日常生活で何か気をつけることがありますか?

① **Are there any other changes I should make in my daily life?**

② **Is there anything else I should do?**

23 ドクター田中

腰を冷やさないでください。お風呂はむしろよいでしょう。何か重いものを持ち上げねばならない時には膝を使うようにして、腰を動かさないようにしてください。

① **Try to keep your lower back warm at all times. Taking a hot bath would be good for that. And when you have to lift something heavy, be sure to use your knees and keep your back straight.**

② **The most important thing is to keep your lower back muscles warm at all times, so hot baths will help. Also, be sure to use your knees for support when you lift something heavy to avoid straining your back.**

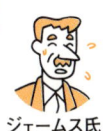

---

24 ジェームス氏

わかりました。
Okay.

---

25 ドクター田中

1週間後の同じ時間にまた来てください。痛みがひどくなったり、何か脚に症状が現れたりしたら連絡してください。来週またお会いしましょう。

① **Come back in a week at the same time. If the pain gets worse, or you have problems with your legs, please call me. See you next week.**

② **In order to monitor your progress, you should come back a week from now. Please don't hesitate to call me before then if the pain gets worse or if it spreads to your legs. See you next week.**

---

26 ジェームス氏

どうもありがとうございました。

① **Thank you very much, Doctor.**

② **I really appreciate your help, Doctor.**

---

27 ドクター田中

どういたしまして。お大事に。

① **Don't mention it. Take care of yourself.**

② **I'm glad I could help, and I hope you feel better soon.**

外科・整形外科用語

あ

アデノイド摘出術	adenoidectomy
胃十二指腸吻合術	gastro-duodenal anastomosis
胃切除術	gastrectomy
打ち身	bruise
O脚	bow-leggedness
錘	weight

か

開胸心臓手術	open heart surgery
回転式フレーム	Stryker frame
外反母趾	bunion
滑車	pulley
関節	joint
関節炎	inflammation of the joint, arthritis
関節強直症	ankylosis
関節固定器	brace
感染創	infected wound
奇形	deformity
義手	artificial arm (hand)
傷跡	scar
義足	artificial leg
ギプス	cast
逆牽引	counter-traction
弓形フレーム	Whitman frame
局所麻酔	local anesthesia
虚弱	weakness
切り傷	cut, wound
筋肉	muscle
筋肉痛	sore muscles
筋膜	fascia
屈曲	flexion
車椅子	wheelchair
けいれん	cramping
腱	tendon
肩甲骨	shoulder blade

	腱鞘炎	tendovaginitis, tenosynovitis
	懸垂牽引	suspension-traction
	拘縮	contraction
	五十肩	frozen shoulder
	骨検診	bone examination
	骨折	fracture
	骨粗鬆症	osteoporosis
	骨盤	pelvis
	骨膜	lamina
	こぶ	bump
	こむらがえり	cramp
	こり	stiffness
	コルセット	corset
さ	鎖骨	collarbone
	坐骨神経痛	hip gout
	痔核切除術	hemorrhoidectomy
	止血鉗子	hemostat
	膝蓋骨	kneecap
	しびれ	numbness
	しもやけ	frostbite
	斜頸	torticollis, wry neck
	銃創	gunshot
	手術室	operating room (OR)
	小手術	minor operation
	消毒／殺菌	disinfection, sterilization
	消毒液	antiseptic solution
	植皮	skin grafting
	靭帯	ligament
	頭蓋骨	skull
	ストッキネット	stockinette
	擦り傷	abrasion
	整復	reduction
	脊椎	spine
	脊椎後彎症	kyphosis

脊椎前彎症	lordosis
脊椎側彎症	scoliosis
切開	incision
切除	excision
切断	amputation
切断後の手足残部	stump
背中の痛み	backpain
全身麻酔	general anesthesia
前立腺切除術	prostatectomy

た

大手術	major operation
大腿骨	femur
大網	major omentum
脱臼	dislocation
脱脂綿	cotton balls
胆嚢切除術	cholecystectomy
虫垂切除術	appendectomy
痛風	gout
突き指	sprained finger
テニス肘	tennis elbow
床ずれ	bedsore

な

内反足	clubfoot
軟骨	cartilage
肉離れ	torn muscle
猫背	humpback
捻挫	sprain

は

絆創膏	adhesive bandage
帆布性の平らなフレーム	Bradford frame
皮下出血	subcutaneous bleeding
引っ掻き傷	scratch
皮膚牽引	skin traction

	副木	splint
	プロテーゼ	prosthesis
	ヘルニア修復術	herniorrhaphy
	扁桃摘出術	tonsillectomy
	扁平足	flatfootedness
	縫合	suture
	包帯	bandage
	包帯を巻く	apply a bandage
	歩行器	walker
ま	松葉杖	crutch
	麻痺	paralysis, palsy
	むち打ち症	whiplash injury
や	やけど	burn
	癒着	adhesion
	腰痛	lower back pain, lumbago
ら	リウマチ	rheumatism
	裂傷	laceration
	肋骨	rib
わ	枠付きフレーム	Balkan frame

Chapter 6 PSYCHIATRY NEUROLOGY

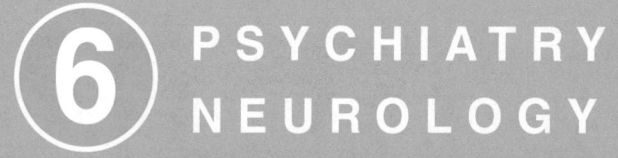

精神・神経科での英会話

What is your major concern?

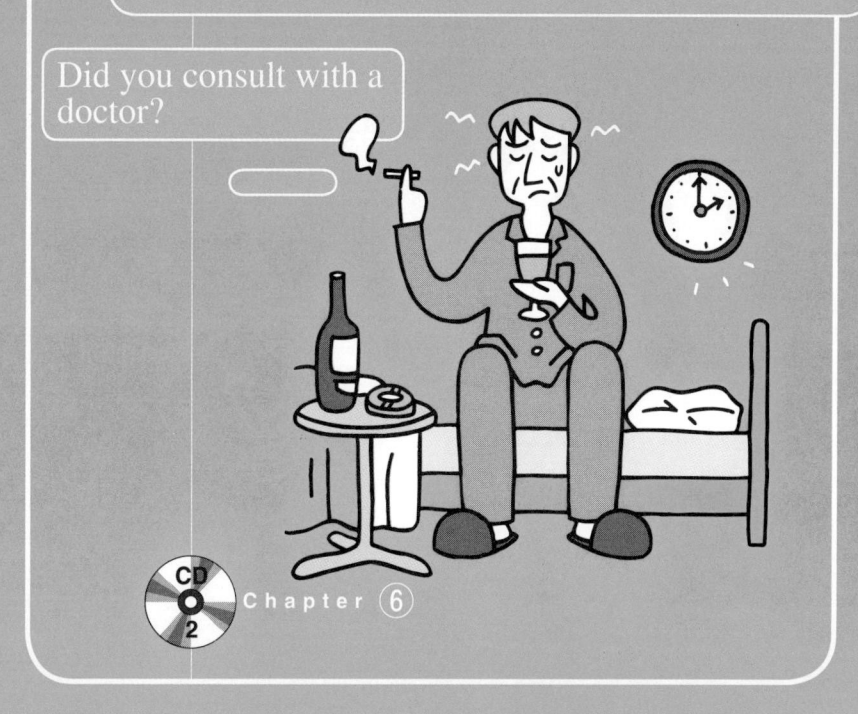

Did you consult with a doctor?

Chapter 6

PSYCHIATRY NEUROLOGY

精神・神経科での英会話

不眠を訴える患者さんの多様な症状に対応します

総合外来では高齢者の方々の約半数が睡眠障害を訴えて来られます。加齢による現象の一つかもしれませんが、精神・神経科には実に様々な症状を訴えて来られる高齢者の方が多いのです。

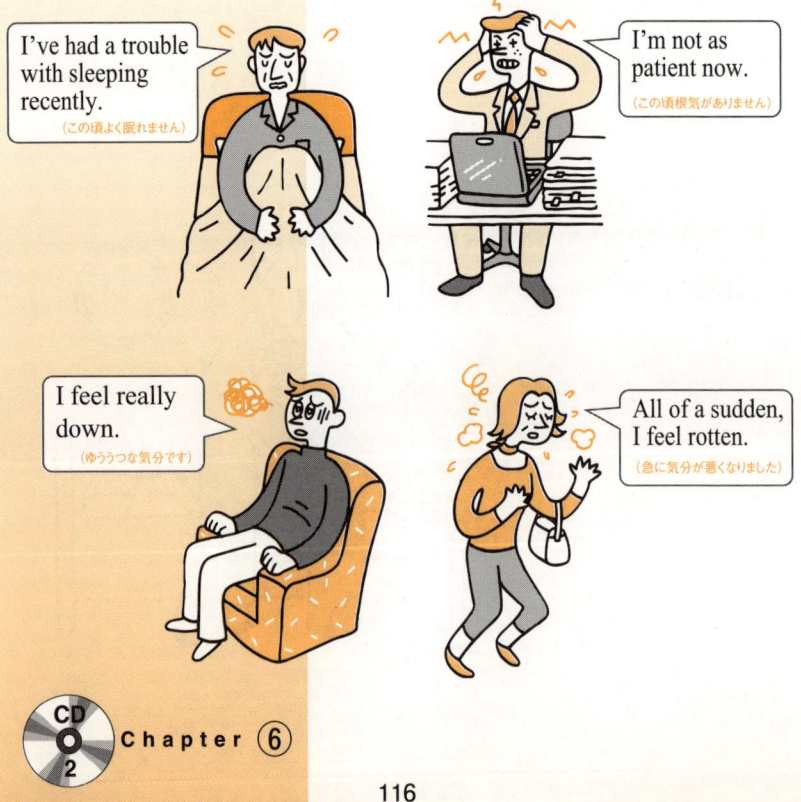

I've had a trouble with sleeping recently.
（この頃よく眠れません）

I'm not as patient now.
（この頃根気がありません）

I feel really down.
（ゆううつな気分です）

All of a sudden, I feel rotten.
（急に気分が悪くなりました）

CD 2　Chapter ⑥

Chapter 6 精神・神経科での英会話

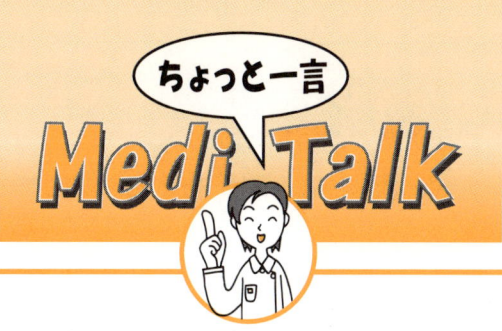

ちょっと一言 Medi Talk

●あなたのいちばんの悩みは何ですか？
What is your major concern?

●寝付きはよいですか？
Do you get to sleep soon?

●何か心配事がありますか？
Do you have anything to worry about?

●音で眠れないのですか？
Does noise often keep you awake at night?

●症状の原因に、何か心当たりはありますか？
Do you know any reason why you have these symptoms?

●医師に相談しましたか？
Did you consult with a doctor?

●睡眠中に怖い夢を見ませんか？
Do you have nightmares while you are sleeping?

ちょっと一言 Medi Talk

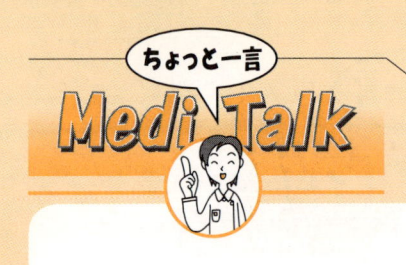

● 人がいないのに、だれかの声が聞こえますか？
① **Do you hear someone's voice in the absence of people?**
② **Do you hear someone's voice when nobody is there?**

● いつも人に見られているように感じますか？
Do you feel that someone is watching you all the time?

● 物事を考えるのに集中できますか？
Are you able to concentrate on something?

● あなたはいつも一人でいるのが好きですか？
Do you like to be alone all the time?

● 気分が落ち込んでいますか？
Have you been feeling depressed?

● 通常の仕事はできていますか？
Have you been able to do regular work?

MediTalk

不眠
Insomnia

Chapter 6 精神・神経科での英会話

ジョンソンさんが、最近、不眠がちになり、田中クリニックを訪れました。

Mr. Johnson visited the Tanaka Clinic, with a complaint of recent insomnia.

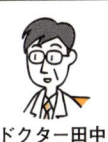

---

1 ドクター田中

どうなさいました?

① What seems to be the trouble?

② What's the problem today?

---

2 ジョンソン氏

この頃よく眠れません。

① I haven't been able to sleep well recently.

② I've had a trouble with sleeping recently.

③ I haven't been sleeping well lately.

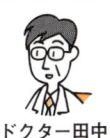

---

3 ドクター田中

最近、あなたの身のまわりに何か大きな変化がありましたか?

① Have you had any serious changes in your life lately?

② Have you experienced any big changes in your life recently?

---

4 ジョンソン氏

特にありません。ただ日本のビジネスにうまく適応できないのですが。

Nothing special, but I still can't adapt myself to the ways of Japanese business.

5 ドクター田中

睡眠環境はどうですか？　騒音に悩まされたりしていませんか？

① How is your sleeping environment? Are you bothered by noise when you're in bed?

② How about your sleeping conditions? Does noise often keep you awake at night?

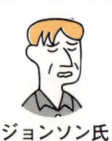

6 ジョンソン氏

いいえ。

No, not really.

7 ドクター田中

あなたの平均的な睡眠のパターンを教えてくれませんか？

① Can you tell me the average pattern of your sleep?

② What's your usual sleep pattern like?

8 ジョンソン氏

ええ。いつも12時に寝ます。しかし、すぐには眠れません。おまけに朝早く目が覚めてしまうことがたびたびあります。

I'm usually in bed by midnight, but I'm not able to get to sleep soon, and to make matters worse, I often wake up too early in the morning.

9 ドクター田中

起きた時、どんな気分ですか？

How do you feel when you wake up?

Chapter 6

精神・神経科での英会話

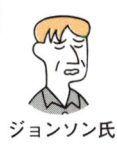

10 ジョンソン氏

よく寝た感じがありません。また、時々ゆううつな気分です。

① I never feel like I've had a good sleep, and sometimes I wake up feeling terribly depressed.

② Sometimes I feel really down, and I never feel well rested.

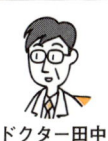

---

11 ドクター田中

最近、気力や意欲の低下はありませんか?

Have you lost any of your energy or your eagerness for work lately?

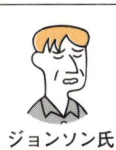

---

12 ジョンソン氏

この頃根気がなく、やる気が起きません。集中力もありません。

① I'm not as patient now, and that hurts my willingness to work. I can't concentrate very well, either.

② My patience is less than before, which makes me not as willing to work, and my concentration has slipped, too.

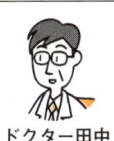

---

13 ドクター田中

それはいけませんね。ところでお酒は飲みますか?

① That's too bad. By the way, do you drink?

② I understand that feeling. By the way, do you drink?

---

14 ジョンソン氏

睡眠不足が心配で毎晩、寝る前に飲まずにいられません。

① I can't stop drinking before going to bed because of the anxiety from the lack of sleep.

② Yes, every night before bed I have a drink, because I'm so worried about insomnia.

15 ドクター田中

運動はしていますか?

① **Do you exercise regularly?**

② **Do you follow any exercise routine?**

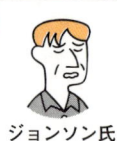

16 ジョンソン氏

残念ながら十分な時間がありません。

① **Unfortunately, I don't have enough time for it.**

② **I'd like to, but I'm just too busy.**

17 ドクター田中

何か夢中になれる趣味はありませんか?

① **Don't you have any hobbies to fill your free time?**

② **Do you pursue any hobbies during your spare time?**

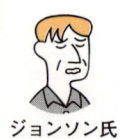

18 ジョンソン氏

特にありません。

Nothing special.

19 ドクター田中

とにかくちょっと検査してみましょう。

① **Anyway, let's have a look at you.**

② **I'd like to examine you now.**

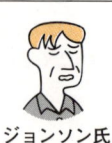

20 ジョンソン氏

はい、先生。

Okay, Doctor.

Chapter 6 精神・神経科での英会話

21 ドクター田中

（検査の後で、ドクター田中はジョンソンさんに説明します）
身体的な異常はないようですね。あなたの不眠は軽いうつ病からきているようです。

You don't seem to have any physical illnesses. I think your insomnia is from the slight depression you've been feeling.

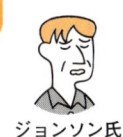

22 ジョンソン氏

うつ病だとは気が付きませんでした。

① **I never thought about the depression by myself.**

② **I never thought that I might be depressed.**

23 ドクター田中

この睡眠薬を夜寝る30分前に1錠、そしてこの抗うつ薬は気分をよくするためのものですから2錠ずつ1日3回飲んでください。そして、1週間後の同じ時間に、また来てください。

Take one of these sleeping tablets 30 minutes before going to bed, and two of these antidepressants three times a day to help you feel better, then come back in a week at the same time.

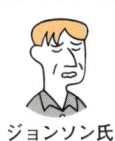

24 ジョンソン氏

この薬には副作用はありませんか？

① **Do these tablets have any side effects?**

② **Are there any side effects?**

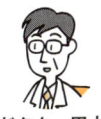

25 ドクター田中

ご心配にはおよびません。この薬の作用は穏やかですから。ただし、アルコールと一緒に飲むのは避けてください。

**No, there's nothing to worry about. These tablets are very mild.
However, please be sure not to take them with alcohol.**

26 ドクター田中

それから寝る前に何か食べたり、コーヒーや紅茶のようなカフェインの入ったものを飲むことは避けてください。

And, please don't have any food or drink containing caffeine, such as coffee or tea before going to bed.

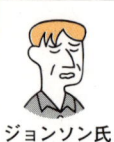

27 ジョンソン氏

わかりました。どうもありがとうございました。

Yes, Doctor, I understand. Thank you very much.

28 ドクター田中

どういたしまして。それでは、また来週。

You're welcome. See you next week.

精神・神経科用語

あ

アルコール依存症	alcoholism
アルツハイマー病	Alzheimer's disease
意識下の	subconscious
意識のある	conscious
うつ病	depression, melancholia
運動性	motor, expressive
落ち着かないこと	restlessness, irritability
温度の知覚	sensitivity to temperature

か

外転足	eversion of foot
過食症	bulimia
かゆい	itching
感覚	sensation
感覚性	sensory, receptive
拮抗運動反復不能症	adiadochokinesis
拒食症	sitophobia, cibophobia
筋緊張	myotonia, muscle tone
筋肉の萎縮	muscle wasting
筋肉のサイズ	muscle size
筋力	muscle strength
けいれん	convulsion
幻覚	hallucination
幻聴	hearing things, auditory hallucination
高所恐怖症	acrophobia
昏睡	coma
昏迷	stupor

さ

錯覚	illusion
指示試験	past-pointing
失行症	apraxia
失語症	aphasia
失神	faint
失認症	amnesia

自閉症	autism
上腕偏位	arm deviation
神経過敏	nervousness
神経衰弱	nervous breakdown, neurasthenia
心身症	psychosomatic disorder
振せん	tremor
振動の知覚	sensitivity to vibration
深部圧迫痛	deep pressure pain
深部感覚テスト	deep sensory test
随意運動	voluntary movements
睡眠障害	sleep disorder
頭軽感	light headedness
頭重感	heavy headedness
精神異常	insanity
精神衰弱	mental deficiency, feeble mindedness
線維束攣縮	fasciculation
譫妄	delirium
躁うつ病	manic-depressive psychosis
躁病	mania

た

大脳神経	cranial nerves
痴愚	imbecile
痴呆症（認知症）	dementia
テタニー	tetany
動悸	palpitation
疼痛のある強直	cramp
鈍	dullness

な

二点識別	two point discrimination
眠気	drowsiness
ノイローゼ	neurosis

は

白痴	idiot
半意識の	semiconscious
ヒステリー	hysteria
表在性瘙痒感	tickling sensation
表在性疼痛	superficial pain
疲労	fatigue
敏感な	sensitive
不安	nervousness
不眠症	insomnia
歩行テスト	gait test
保続症	perseveration

ま

麻痺する	paralyze
麻薬中毒	narcotic addiction
無意識	unconscious
めまい	vertigo, dizziness
妄想	delusion
物忘れ	forgetfulness

や

薬物乱用	substance abuse
抑うつ病	depression

ら

立体認識不能症	astereognosis
れん縮	spasm
魯鈍	moron, stupid
ロンベルグテスト	Romberg walk in tandem

Chapter 7 PEDIATRICS

小児科での英会話

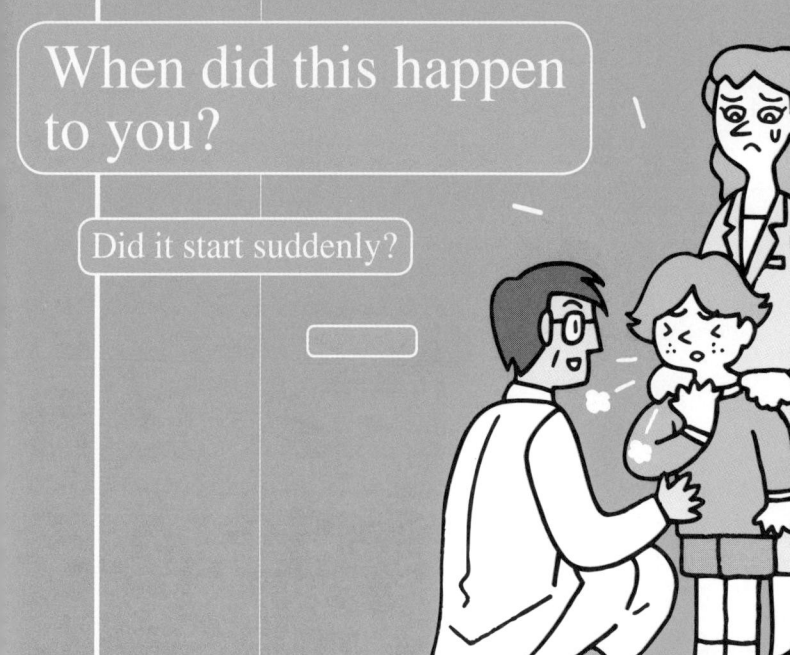

When did this happen to you?

Did it start suddenly?

Chapter 7

Chapter 7 PEDIATRICS
小児科での英会話

風邪やアレルギー症状が小児に多い疾患です

小児の病気といえば、風邪や腹部の病気がいちばん多いようです。そのほか、小児気管支喘息やいろいろなアレルギー症状を起こして受診するケースが多く見られます。

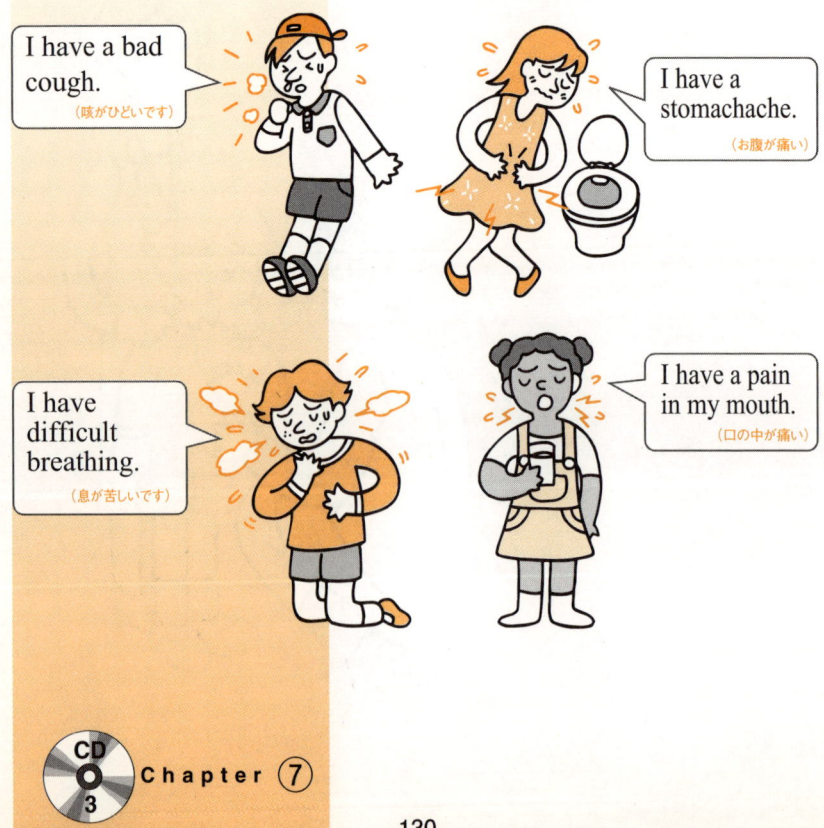

I have a bad cough.
（咳がひどいです）

I have a stomachache.
（お腹が痛い）

I have difficult breathing.
（息が苦しいです）

I have a pain in my mouth.
（口の中が痛い）

CD 3 Chapter ⑦

Chapter 7 小児科での英会話

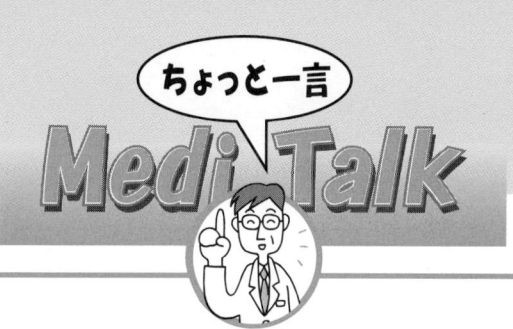

ちょっと一言 Medi Talk

● 症状が起きたのはいつですか？
When did this happen to you?

● 以前にも咳き込んだことはありますか？
Has he (she) had wheezing before?

● 突然、咳き込み始めたのですか？
Did it start suddenly?

● 咳が始まったきっかけは何ですか？
What started the wheezing?

運動ですか？
Exercise?

冷たい空気にあたったのですか？
Cold air?

ほこりでしょうか？
Dust?

風邪をひきましたか？
Does he (she) have a cold?

気が動転していましたか？
Was he (she) upset?

犬や猫でしょうか？
Dogs or cats?

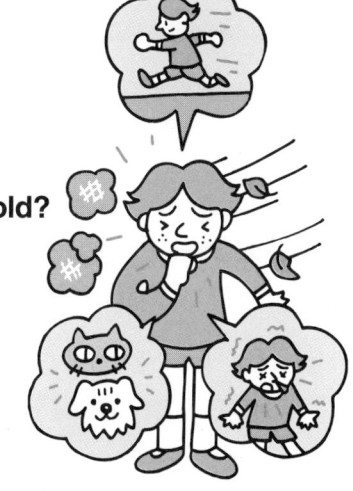

Medi Talk
ちょっと一言

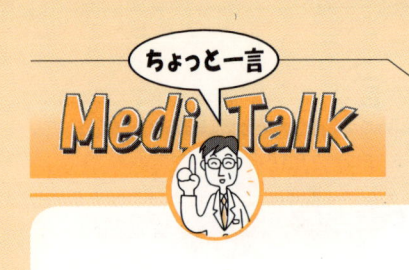

● 嘔吐しましたか？
Has he (she) been vomiting?

● 熱はありましたか？
Has he (she) had a fever?

● アレルギーはありますか？
Does he (she) have allergies?

● 発疹はありますか？
Does he (she) have a rash?

● 家族の中でアレルギーのある方はいらっしゃいますか？
Does anyone else in the family have allergies?

● 嘔吐が続く場合はご連絡ください。連絡先は〇〇〇〇です。
Please call if he (she) continues to vomit. The phone number is 〇〇〇〇.

● 呼吸が苦しいようなら私どもへご連絡ください。
Please call us if he (she) continues to have difficult breathing.

● 水分を十分に与えてください。
Give him (her) lots of fluids.

Chapter 7　小児科での英会話

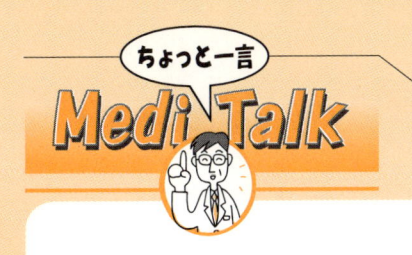

ちょっと一言 Medi Talk

●今夜は病院で様子を見ましょう。
Your child must stay in the hospital tonight.

●何か変わった様子はありませんか？
Has he (she) had changes in his (her) behavior?

機嫌が悪い
irritable

食欲がない
poor feeding

咳
cough

遊びたがらない
not playful

発疹が出ている
any rash

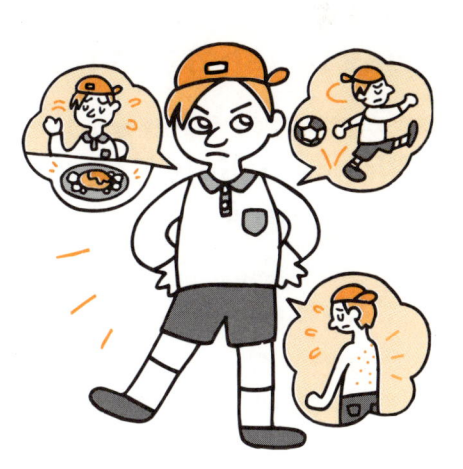

●熱はありませんか？
Does he (she) have a fever?

●下痢や嘔吐はどうですか？
Has he (she) had diarrhea or vomiting?

ちょっと一言 Medi Talk

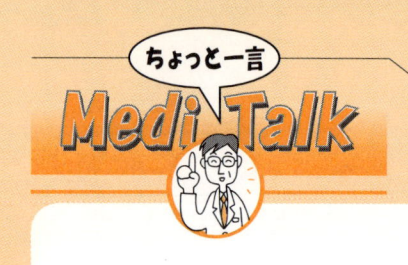

● 食事に関係なく嘔吐しますか、それとも食事をした時だけですか？
Is he (she) vomiting all the time or only when he (she) eats?

● 便は水のようですか、それとも柔らかい便ですか？
Is the stool watery or just soft?

● 予防接種はすみましたか？
Has he (she) had inoculations?

● 次の症状が続くようなら連絡してください。
Please call us if the following symptoms continue.

> 熱が下がらない。
> **His (her) temperature doesn't go down.**
>
> 嘔吐が続く。
> **He (she) continues to vomit.**
>
> 下痢がひどくなる。
> **The diarrhea worsens.**
>
> 呼吸が苦しそう。
> **He (she) has difficult breathing.**
>
> 水分をとらない。
> **He (she) doesn't want to drink.**

MediTalk

小児気管支喘息
Child asthmatic bronchitis

Chapter **7**
小児科での英会話

ドワイヤー夫人が息子のマーク君を連れて、田中クリニックを訪れました。

Mrs. Dwyer visited the Tanaka Clinic, with her son Mark.

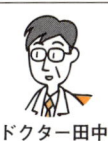

---

1 ドクター田中

こんにちは。今日はどうしましたか?

Hello, what's the matter today?

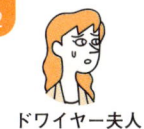

---

2 ドワイヤー夫人

昨夜マークが喘息発作を起こして眠れなかったのでまいりました。

① **I brought Mark here because he had an asthmatic attack and couldn't sleep last night.**

② **My son, Mark, couldn't sleep at all last night due to an asthmatic attack, so I brought him here for treatment.**

---

3 ドクター田中

発作のとき、ふだんはどうしていますか?

① **What do you usually do when he has attacks?**

② **What kind of treatment does he usually receive when he has attacks?**

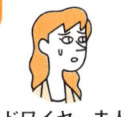

---

4 ドワイヤー夫人

昼は近所の医院、夜の場合は救急病院で吸入をしてもらいます。

① **I take him to a clinic near my house in the daytime, and when it happens at night, I take him to an emergency hospital for inhalation.**

② **Either I take him to a nearby clinic for inhalation in the daytime, or to an emergency hospital if it happens at night.**

5 ドクター田中

今回は、どうして私どもの病院にいらしたのですか？

Why did you come here today?

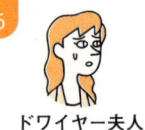

6 ドワイヤー夫人

再び起こると思っていなかった発作が昨夜起こったので、とても驚いたからです。

① I came here today because I never expected an attack like that would happen again, and it really scared me last night.

② I didn't expect he would have another attack like that, and it made me worried.

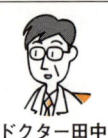

7 ドクター田中

今までに点滴や入院の経験はありますか？ お子さんの喘息がいちばんひどかったのは、何歳くらいの時ですか？

Has he ever stayed in a hospital, or been given an intravenous (IV) drip infusion? How old was he when the symptoms were the worst?

8 ドワイヤー夫人

3〜4歳の時ですが、いつも吸入で治りました。

He was about three or four, but usually the inhalations helped him get well at that time.

9 ドクター田中

発作を起こしていない時は、何か治療を受けましたか？

① Was he treated for asthma when he didn't have attacks?

② Did he receive treatment for asthma when he didn't have attacks?

Chapter 7 小児科での英会話

10 ドワイヤー夫人

ひどかった頃、1年間くらい予防薬を飲んでいましたが、今は何もしていません。

① He took medicine for prevention of asthma for a year when he had the most violent attacks, but he isn't taking anything now.

② He isn't taking anything now, but when the asthma was severe, he took asthma prevention medicine for a year.

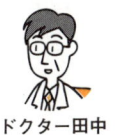

11 ドクター田中

喘息で苦しい時は、マーク君、君は大きな声を出したり泣いたりするの?

① Mark, do you shout or cry when you suffer from the attacks?

② Mark, do the asthmatic attacks make you shout or cry?

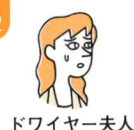

12 ドワイヤー夫人

……そうなのです。いつも騒いで大変なのです。

① ..... Yes, he does. He causes an awful disturbance.

② ..... Yes, Doctor, they do. He makes quite a lot of noise.

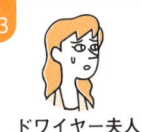

13 ドワイヤー夫人

息が苦しい時に大声を出すと、もっと苦しくなってきます。そうでしょう、マーク。

① If you shout when you're out of breath, your breathing gets more difficult, doesn't it, Mark?

② It's harder to breathe if you shout when you're out of breath, isn't it, Mark?

14 マーク君

はい。

I think so.

15 ドクター田中

（マーク君に向かって）
これからは発作の時、泣いたり騒いだりしないこと。吸入で治る発作はたいてい自分で治せますからね。

Don't cry and shout after this when you have attacks. You can make the attacks go away by yourself, because you don't have such a serious case if they can be stopped by inhalation.

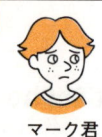

16 マーク君

…………。

……… Umm.

17 ドワイヤー夫人

どうすれば治るのですか？

① What can we do to cure him of this?
② How can he be cured?

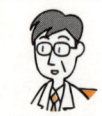

18 ドクター田中

腹式呼吸をすること、毎日水分を十分とって痰を上手に出すこと、発作止めの薬を飲むこと、などです。

You should help him do abdominal breathing, give him plenty of liquid everyday to get rid of the phlegm, give him medicine to stop the attacks, and so on.

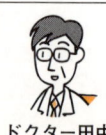

19 ドクター田中

今日はこれから、アレルギーの血液検査と、腹式呼吸、痰を上手に出す練習を始めましょう。

Today, I'm going to do a blood test to check for allergies, let him practice abdominal breathing, and show him how to get rid of phlegm.

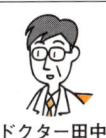

---

20 ドクター田中

4歳くらいの子供でも、できるようになりますよ。

① **It's easy even for a four-year-old child.**

② **Even a four-year-old child can do it!**

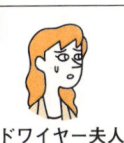

---

21 ドワイヤー夫人

発作止めの薬は、どのように飲むのでしょうか？

How should he take the medicine to stop the attacks?

---

22 ドクター田中

6時間以上の間隔をあけてください。効果が出るには1〜2時間かかります。

① **The medicine should be taken at six hours interval at least. It's effect will be felt one to two hours after taking it.**

② **The medicine takes effect between one and two hours after ingestion, so he should let at least six hours pass before taking it again.**

---

23 ドクター田中

来週のアレルギー外来で、血液検査の結果と日常生活の注意などをお話ししましょう。

I'll give you the results of the blood test, along with some advice on what to be careful about Mark's daily life when we meet next week in the allergy outpatient clinic.

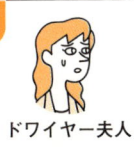

---

24 ドワイヤー夫人

では、来週うかがいます。ありがとうございました。

So, I'll see you here next week. Thank you.

MediTalk

小児科疾患（ヘルペス）
Pediatric disease (Herpes zoster)

ウイリアムス夫人が娘のベスを連れて田中クリニックを訪れました。

Mrs. Williams visited the Tanaka Clinic, with her daughter Beth.

---

1 ドクター田中

どうなさいましたか？

What's the matter with her?

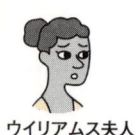

---

2 ウイリアムス夫人

娘のベスが1週間前から38℃以上の熱を出して、食事をとらなくなったのです。

① **My daughter, Beth, has had a high fever 38℃, and hasn't had any meals for one week.**

② **For about a week now, my daughter Beth has been suffering from a fever of more than 38℃, along with a total loss of appetite.**

---

3 ドクター田中

咳は出ますか？

① **Does she have a cough?**

② **Has she been coughing?**

---

4 ウイリアムス夫人

特に出ません。

① **Not particularly.**

② **Not that I've noticed.**

---

5 ドクター田中

嘔吐や下痢など、何かお腹の症状はありますか？

① **Does she have any stomach symptoms, for example, an upset stomach, or diarrhea?**

Chapter 7

小児科での英会話

② How about an upset stomach, or diarrhea?

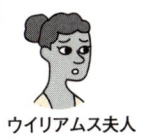

6 ウイリアムス夫人

特別ありませんが、とにかく食べることを嫌がります。

① Not really, but she still doesn't have any desire to eat.

② No, neither one, yet she simply has no interest in eating whatsoever.

7 ドクター田中

水分は1日どのくらいとりますか?

How much water does she drink a day?

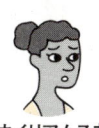

8 ウイリアムス夫人

口の中が痛いようで、昨日は牛乳2本分くらいしか飲みませんでした。

She seems to have some pain in her mouth, so she drank only two milk bottles of water yesterday.

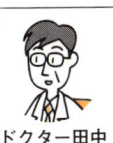

9 ドクター田中

だいぶ少ないですね。それでは尿の回数はどうですか?

① It's such a small amount. And how often does she urinate?

② It's not nearly enough. And how often has she been urinating?

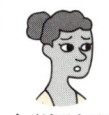

10 ウイリアムス夫人

少なくなっていますが、今朝は排尿がありました。

① The frequency has been decreasing, but fortunately she urinated this morning.

② Not as often as usual, but luckily she did go this morning.

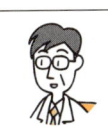

11 ドクター田中

それでは診察をしましょうネ、ベスちゃん。

① Well, I'd like to examine you now, Beth.

② Okay, Beth, it's time for me to examine you.

12 ナース/石田

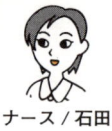

お洋服を脱がせて、ベッドの上に寝かせてください。

① Would you please take Beth's clothes off, and lay her down on the examining table?

② Would you please remove her clothes, and have her lie down on the examining table?

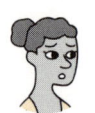

---

13 ウイリアムス夫人

（ベスちゃんを診察した後、ウイリアムス夫人がドクター田中に向かって尋ねます）
どんな具合でしょうか？

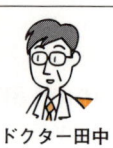

How is she?

---

14 ドクター田中

お嬢さんは、単純ヘルペスというウイルス性の感染症です。

① She has herpes simplex, which is a kind of viral infection.

② Your daughter has a form of viral infection known as herpes simplex.

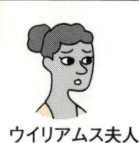

---

15 ウイリアムス夫人

それはどういう病気でしょうか？　重い病気なのですか？

① What kind of disease is it? Do you think it's anything serious?

② I don't know anything about it. Is it dangerous?

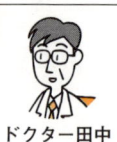

---

16 ドクター田中

発熱が長期にわたることがありますが、重い病気ではありません。そろそろ熱が下がってくると思います。

It causes a fever which lasts for quite a while, but it's not a serious disease. I think that her fever will go down soon.

Chapter 7 小児科での英会話

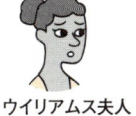

17 ウイリアムス夫人

安心しました。何か気を付けることはありますか?

① I'm relieved to hear that. What should I do to help her feel better?

② That's a relief. How should I take care of her at home?

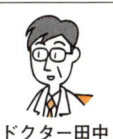

18 ドクター田中

水分を十分に与えてください。お口の中が痛くなる病気なので、刺激のない柔らかい食べ物を十分与えてあげてください。

① Feed her a lot of liquids. Herpes simplex also causes painful sores in the mouth, so you should feed her bland soft food.

② Make sure she drinks plenty of liquids, and feed her mild, soft food, so it won't irritate the sores in her mouth, which are caused by the disease.

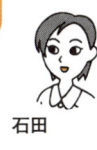

19 石田

もし今よりも飲めなくなってぐったりするようなら、いつでもご相談ください。

① If she can't drink any more than what she drinks now, or if she starts to feel more lethargic, please call me.

② Give me a call if she feels even less energetic than now, or if she's unable to drink more than she has been.

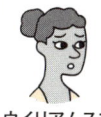

20 ウイリアムス夫人

ありがとうございました。

① Thank you very much.

② I really appreciate it.

小児科用語

あ

浅い	shallow
あせも	heat rash
うずくまる	squat
腋窩の（で）	axillary, by axilla
黄疸	jaundice
おたふく風邪	mumps

か

寛解、軽減	lysis
間欠熱	intermittent fever
危機	crisis
吸気	inspiration, inhalation
クスマウル呼吸	Kussmaul respiration
口蓋裂	cleft palate
口腔の（で）	oral, by mouth
口唇裂	harelip
肛門の（で）	rectal, by rectum
呼気	expiration
呼吸	respiration
呼吸器	respirator
呼吸困難	shortness of breath, dyspnea

さ

酸素吸入（テント）	oxygen inhalation
自家中毒	autointoxication
持続熱	continuous fever
弛張熱	remittent fever
ジフテリア	diphtheria
斜視	strabismus
出生後に	postnatally
猩紅熱	scarlet fever
心雑音	heart murmur
心室中隔欠損	ventricular septal defect (VSD)
心房中隔欠損	atrial septal defect (ASD)
水頭症	water baby
仙痛	colic

Chapter 7 小児科での英会話

	先天性心臓血管奇形	congenital cardiovascular anomalies
	早産児	premature baby

た	体温	body temperature
	体温計	thermometer
	ダウン症候群	Down's syndrome
	チアノーゼ	cyanosis
	チェーン・ストークス呼吸	Cheyne-Stokes respiration
	中耳炎	inflammation of the middle ear
	中枢神経系統	CNS (central nervous system)
	徴候	episode
	動脈管開存症	PDA (patent ductus arteriosus)

な	難聴	impaired hearing
	乳幼児突然死症候群	SIDS (sudden infant death syndrome)
	熱	fever

は	はしか	measles
	破傷風	tetanus
	BCG	BCG (Bacillus Calmette-Guérin)
	鼻炎	inflammation of the nose
	百日咳	whooping cough
	ファロー四徴症	tetralogy of Fallot
	風疹	rubella, German measles
	深い	deep
	扁桃炎	tonsillitis
	ポリオ	polio

ま	水疱瘡	chicken pox
	無呼吸	apnea

や・ら

夜泣き　　　　　　　night cry

リウマチ熱　　　　　rheumatic fever

Chapter 8 GYNECOLOGY

婦人科での英会話

When was your last delivery?

Are you on the pill?

Chapter 8

Chapter 8
GYNECOLOGY
婦人科での英会話

不正出血は、婦人科で特に多い症状です

婦人科を訪れる方々には様々な訴えがありますが、まず多いのが、不正出血でしょう。中年になると、必ず直面する問題だと思います。

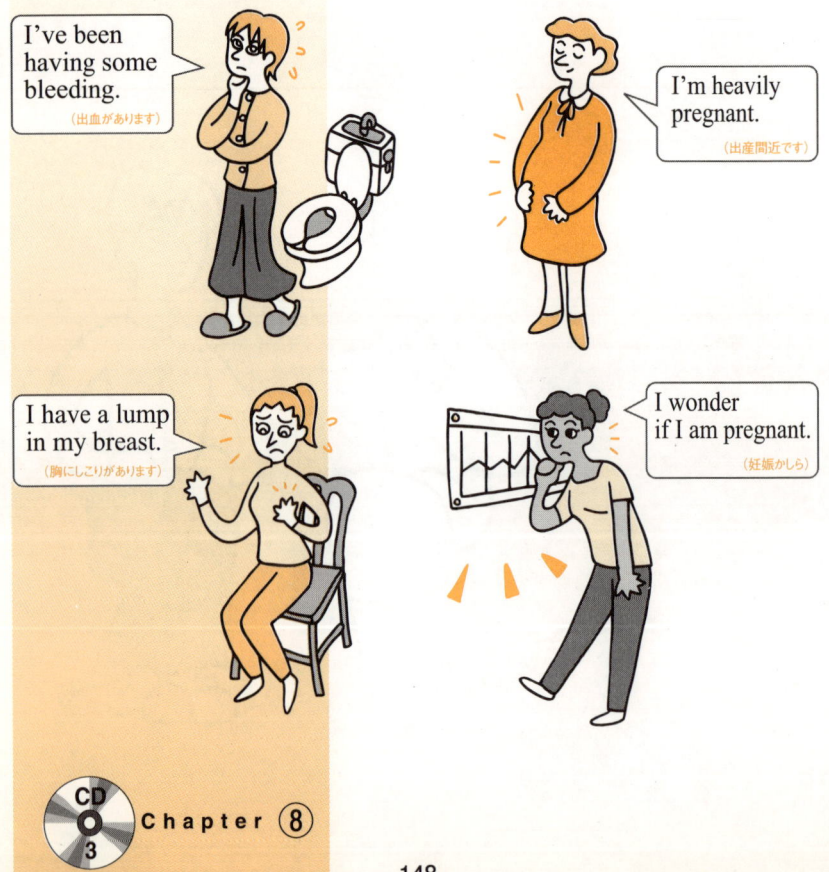

I've been having some bleeding.
（出血があります）

I'm heavily pregnant.
（出産間近です）

I have a lump in my breast.
（胸にしこりがあります）

I wonder if I am pregnant.
（妊娠かしら）

CD 3 Chapter 8

ちょっと一言 Medi Talk

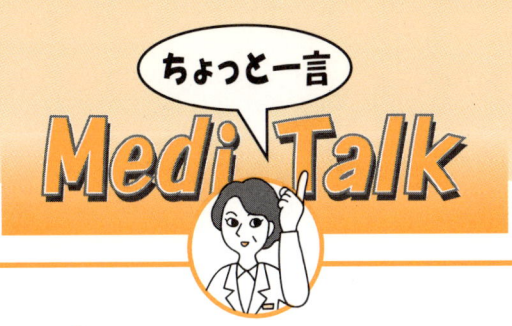

Chapter 8 婦人科での英会話

● 生理は順調ですか？
How about your periods, are they regular?

● 最後の生理はいつでしたか？
When was your last period?

● 不正出血やおりものがありますか？
Do you have any vaginal bleeding or discharge?

● 妊娠なさっていますか？
Are you pregnant?

● お子さんは何人いらっしゃいますか？
How many children do you have?

● 最後の出産はいつでしたか？
When was your last delivery?

● 流産されたことはありますか？
Have you had any miscarriages?

● 分娩の際、合併症を起こしましたか？
Did you have any complications with your deliveries?

Medi Talk ちょっと一言

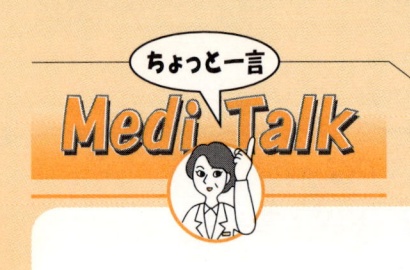

●お子さんは母乳で育てましたか？
Did you breast-feed your children?

●ピルを飲んでいますか？
Are you on the pill?

●何か避妊をされていますか？
Do you use any birth control?

●乳房にしこりができたことがありますか？
Have you ever noticed a mass in your breasts?

●乳汁の異常な分泌がありますか？
Do you have abnormal discharge from your nipples?

●以前にも婦人科疾患にかかったことがありますか？
Have you ever had a gynecologic disease?

●このガウンを着てください。
Please put on this gown.

●深呼吸をしてください。
Breathe deeply.

MediTalk

不正出血 / Irregular bleeding

Chapter 8 婦人科での英会話

テイラー夫人が、最近、不正出血が出るようになり田中クリニックを訪れました。

Ms. Taylor visited the Tanaka Clinic, because of irregular bleeding which developed recently.

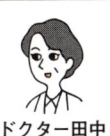

---

1 ドクター田中

どうしましたか？

What can I do for you?

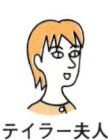

---

2 テイラー夫人

時々出血があるのですが。

① **I've been having some bleeding occasionally.**

② **Sometimes I suffer from bleeding.**

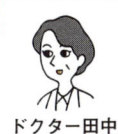

---

3 ドクター田中

どんな時に出血しますか？

① **When does the bleeding occur?**

② **When does it usually happen?**

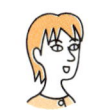

---

4 テイラー夫人

生理が終わった後、少したってから出血があります。

① **It comes after my menstrual period finishes.**

② **Once my period ends, the bleeding starts.**

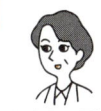

---

5 ドクター田中

そういう出血はたびたびあるのですか？

① **How often does the bleeding appear?**

② **Can you tell me the frequency of the bleeding?**

151

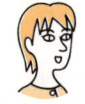

6 テイラー夫人
6か月くらい前から時々あります。癌が心配なのですが。
I've had it periodically for the last six months. I'm worried that maybe I have cancer.

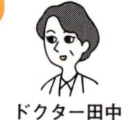

7 ドクター田中
今までに婦人科の診察、あるいは癌の検査を受けたことがありますか?
Have you ever consulted a gynecologist or been tested for cancer?

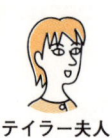

8 テイラー夫人
まだ、一度もありません。
① **No, I've never done either one.**
② **No, this is my first time for both.**

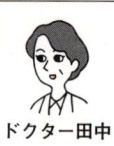

9 ドクター田中
それでは診察の後、癌の検査をしてみましょう。
① **Well, I'll examine you, and after that I'll do a cancer test.**
② **Well, I'll take a look at you now, then we'll check for cancer.**

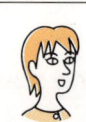

10 テイラー夫人
お願いします。
① **All right.**
② **That sounds fine.**

Chapter 8 婦人科での英会話

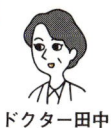

11 ドクター田中

内診台に上がってください。
Please get onto the gynecological stand.

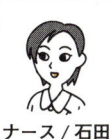

12 ナース／石田

できるだけ力を抜いて楽にしてください。
① **Try to relax as completely as you can.**
② **Please relax as much as possible.**

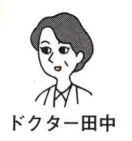

13 ドクター田中

（ドクター田中は、テイラー夫人を診察した後）
内診では子宮や卵巣には、特に異常は認められません。
① **There's nothing abnormal about your uterus or your ovaries.**
② **Your uterus and ovaries don't seem to have anything wrong with them.**

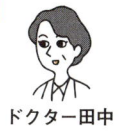

14 ドクター田中

いちばんに考えられるのはホルモン異常による出血ですが、癌の心配をなくすために細胞を詳しく検査してみます。
I think that the bleeding comes from a hormonal disorder, but to ease your anxiety about cancer, I'll test some of your cells to see if they're cancerous or not.

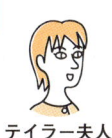

15 テイラー夫人

出血はこのままにしておいてよいでしょうか？
① **Isn't there some kind of treatment you can give me to stop the bleeding?**
② **Can't you do something to make the bleeding stop?**

16. ドクター田中

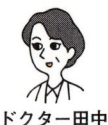

あまり心配しないでください。ホルモン性の出血だと思いますので、注射で止めましょう。

Try not to worry too much about it. As I mentioned before, your condition is due to a hormonal problem, so I'll give you an injection to stop the bleeding.

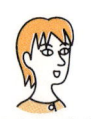

17. テイラー夫人

今度はいつ受診したらよいでしょうか?

① When should I come to see you next?

② When would you like me to come back?

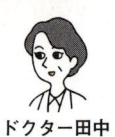

18. ドクター田中

細胞検査の結果が1週間以内に出るので来週受診してください。

① Please come back next week. I'll tell you the results of the test then.

② I'd like you to make an appointment for next week. I'll tell you the results of the test then.

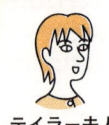

19. テイラー夫人

今度来る時まで、何か注意することはありますか?

① Is there anything special I need to do until my next visit?

② Between now and then, do I need to do anything special?

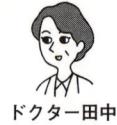

20. ドクター田中

出血がこれ以上増えなければ、普通の日常生活で結構です。

① No, you can continue to live as you normally do as long as the bleeding doesn't increase.

② No. Following your regular lifestyle will be fine, as long as there is no increase in the bleeding.

産婦人科用語

あ

安全ピン	safety pin
育児室	nursery
色	color
会陰	perineum
会陰縫合	repair (of perineum)
横位	transverse or lateral position
おむつ	diaper, nappy
悪露	leucorrhea, lochia

か

外陰の清拭	perineal care
吃逆	hiccup, hiccough
吸引器	suction
経産婦	multipara
血球の塊	clot
月経	menstruation
月経過多	profuse menstruation
月経間出血	intermenstrual bleeding
月経困難	dysmenorrhea
更年期障害	menopausal disorder
骨盤	pelvis
骨盤位	breech

さ

最終月経日	date of last menstrual period
臍帯	cord, umbilical cord
臍帯鉗子	cord clamp
産科鉗子	delivery forceps
産褥	puerperium
産前の合併症	prenatal complications
子癇	eclampsia, toxemia of pregnancy
子宮	uterus
子宮外妊娠	ectopic pregnancy
子宮癌	uterine cancer
子宮筋腫	uterine myoma

子宮頸部	cervix
子宮口開大	dilatation of cervix
子宮底部	fundus of uterus
子宮内膜症	endometriosis
子宮内膜搔爬術	dilating and curettage (D&C)
死産	still birth
自然分娩	spontaneous delivery
周期	cycle
収縮	contraction
準備室	preparation room
症状	symptom(s)
初産婦	primipara
初潮	onset
人工栄養	bottle feeding, formula
新生児	new born, infant
陣痛	labor
陣痛室	labor room
陣痛促進	induction of labor
寝籠	bassinet
性質	character
正常な	regular
前置胎盤	placenta previa
早産	premature birth
側切開	episiotomy
蘇生	resuscitation

た

胎位	presentation
胎向	position
胎児心音	fetal heart sound
胎児心音聴診器	fetoscope
胎動	fetal movement, quickening
胎盤	placenta
膣	vagina
膣部消失	effacement
帝王切開	cesarean section

	頭位	vertex
な	ナプキン	napkin
	乳癌	breast cancer
	乳腺炎	inflammation of the mammary gland
	乳頭	nipple
	乳房	breasts
	妊娠	pregnancy
	妊娠期間	duration of pregnancy
	妊娠終了の型	type of termination of pregnancy
	妊娠線	striations of pregnancy
	妊娠中絶	therapeutic abortion, artificial abortion
	妊娠中毒症	toxicosis of pregnancy
	妊娠の終了	termination of pregnancy
は	破水	rupture of membrane
	初胎動	quickening
	パパニコロー染色	Papanicolaou's stain
	反芻	regurgitation
	不快感	discomfort
	腹部圧痛	abdominal tenderness
	婦人科的診察	gynecological examination
	不正な	irregular
	分娩期	duration of labor
	分娩室	delivery room
	閉経期	menopause
	閉経後の性器出血	bleeding since menopause
	保温器	incubator
	哺乳ビン	feeding bottle

ま		
	未熟児	premature baby

ら		
	卵管	salpinx, fallopian tube
	卵巣	ovaries
	卵巣炎	oophoritis
	流産	abortion, miscarriage

Chapter 9 DERMATOLOGY

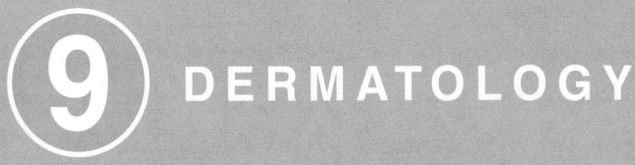

皮膚科での英会話

How long have you had the rash?

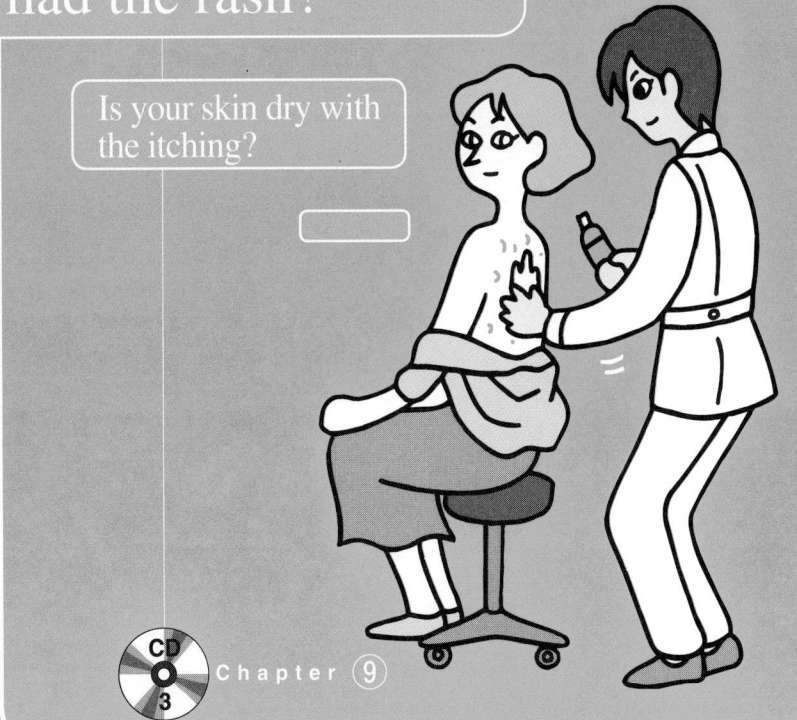

Is your skin dry with the itching?

Chapter 9

Chapter 9
DERMATOLOGY
皮膚科での英会話

皮膚科の症状は非常にバラエティに富んでいます

皮膚科の疾患にも急性のものから、慢性のものまで、様々な病型があります。症状がいちばん多岐にわたる分野かもしれません。

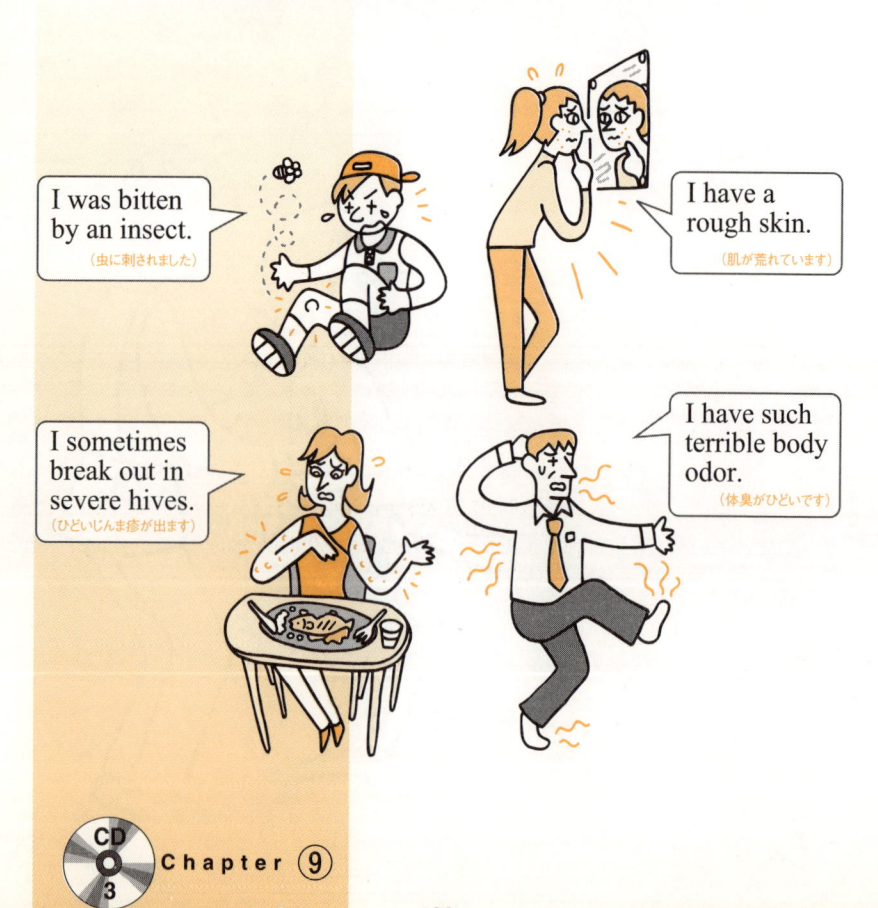

I was bitten by an insect.
（虫に刺されました）

I have a rough skin.
（肌が荒れています）

I sometimes break out in severe hives.
（ひどいじんま疹が出ます）

I have such terrible body odor.
（体臭がひどいです）

CD 3 Chapter 9

Chapter 9 皮膚科での英会話

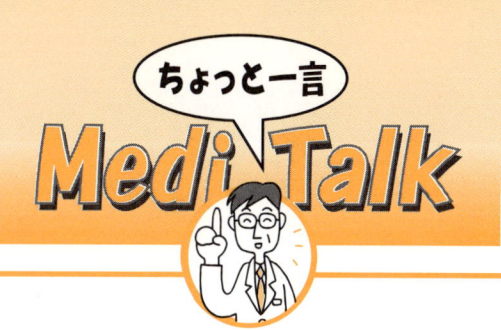

Medi Talk — ちょっと一言

- 喘息、花粉症や薬物過敏によるアレルギーを起こしたことはありませんか？

  Have you ever had asthma, hay fever, or an allergy caused by sensitivity for medicines?

- 発疹はどのくらい出ていますか？

  How long have you had the rash?

- 漆にかぶれたことはありますか？

  Have you ever had any reaction to poison ivy?

- 虫に刺されましたか？

  Has an insect bitten you?

- 皮膚の色の変化や、異常な発汗に気付いたことはありませんか？

  Have you noticed any changes of skin color or abnormal sweating?

- 毛髪の生えかたや、性質はどうですか？

  How about your hair distribution and its character?

ちょっと一言 Medi Talk

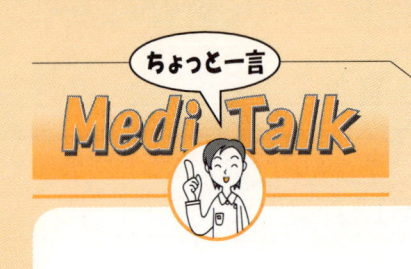

●爪はどうですか、何か変わったことはありませんか？
How about your nails, have you ever noticed any changes?

●皮膚が乾燥してかゆみがありませんか？
Is your skin dry with the itching?

●何かいつもと違うものを食べませんでしたか？
Have you eaten anything different lately?

●最近、いつもとは違う新しい石鹸を使いませんでしたか？
Have you used a new soap lately for yourself?

●洗剤を変えませんでしたか？
Have you used a new detergent for your clothes?

●靴は足に合っていますか？
Do your shoes fit well?

●魚を食べて、じんま疹が出たことがありますか？
Have you ever had the hives when you eat fish?

MediTalk

発疹・湿疹

Rash

Chapter **9**

皮膚科での英会話

メーソンさんが、腕の発疹のことで田中クリニックに相談にきました。

Ms. Mason visited the Tanaka Clinic because of rashes on her arm.

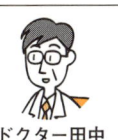

---

1 ドクター田中

お待たせしてすみません。どうなさいましたか?

I'm sorry to have kept you waiting. What can I do for you today?

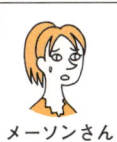

---

2 メーソンさん

腕輪をつけると、いつも皮膚に発疹が出ます。

① **Whenever I wear a wrist band, my skin breaks out in a rash.**

② **I've got a problem with rashes when my skin comes into contact with the wrist band I wear.**

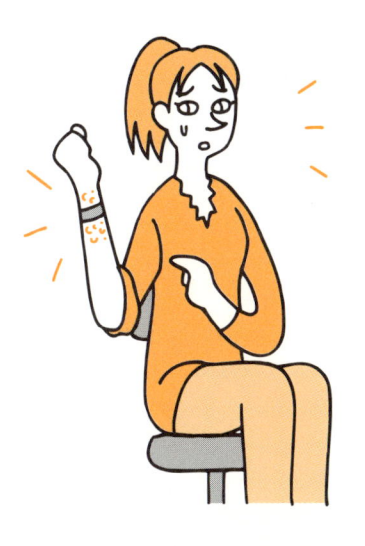

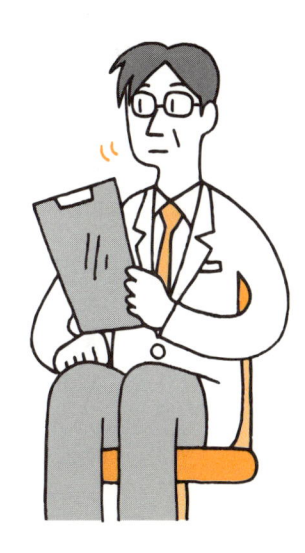

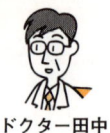

3 ドクター田中
かゆみはありますか？ ほかの場所に発疹は出ますか？
Is it itchy? Where else do you have the rash?

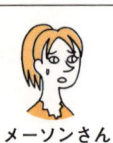

4 メーソンさん
ええ、かゆいですが、ほかのところには出ていません。
Yes, it is itchy, but I don't have it anywhere else.

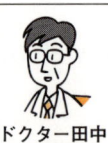

5 ドクター田中
それでは、抗ヒスタミン剤をお出ししましょう。その腕輪はつけないようにするか、直接肌に触れないようにしてください。
I will give you antihistamines. Do not wear the wrist band and avoid direct contact with it.

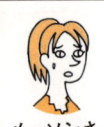

6 メーソンさん
わかりました。
I see, Doctor.

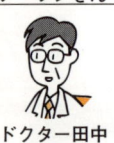

7 ドクター田中
アレルギーの検査を受けたことはありますか？
Have you ever been tested for allergies?

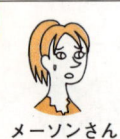

8 メーソンさん
受けていないので、検査していただけますか。
No, not yet. So, I'd like to be tested.

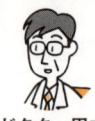

9 ドクター田中
わかりました。では、受付で予約をしてください。
All right. Make an appointment to test for allergies at the receptionist's counter.

MediTalk

体臭
Body odor

Chapter 9
皮膚科での英会話

ペイジ氏は、体臭がひどくて、田中クリニックを訪れました。

Mr. Page visited the Tanaka Clinic because he has terrible body odor.

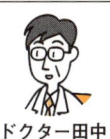

---

1 ドクター田中

どうされました?

① What seems to be the trouble?

② How can I help you today?

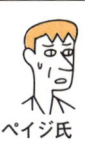

---

2 ペイジ氏

体臭がひどいのですが、何か止めるためのいい方法はありませんか?

① I have such a terrible body odor. Could you tell me a good way to stop it?

② Please help me get rid of my horrible body odor.

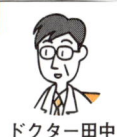

---

3 ドクター田中

毎日、皮膚を清潔に保つことが大切ですが、市販薬の消臭剤を使ってください。

It is important to keep your skin clean, however, you can also use a deodorant. You can get it at any pharmacy.

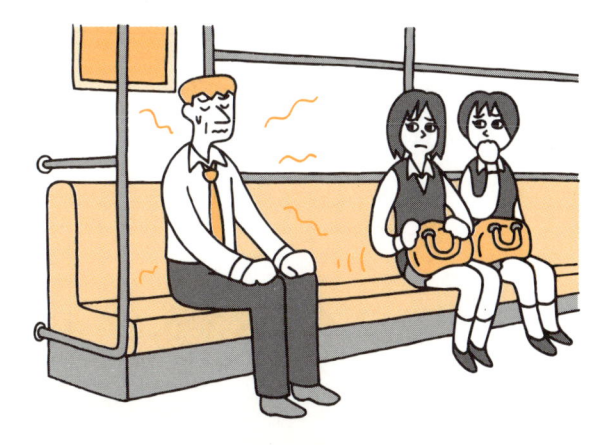

MediTalk

水虫 / Athlete's foot

水虫に悩まされているマーヴィン氏が田中クリニックを訪れました。

Mr. Marvin visited the Tanaka Clinic because of athlete's foot.

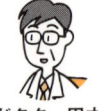

1 ドクター田中

どうされました?

① What seems to be the trouble?

② How can I help you today?

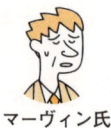

2 マーヴィン氏

先月から水虫に悩まされていまして、かゆくてたまりません。

① I've been suffering from a terrible case of athlete's foot since last month. The itching is just unbearable.

② I've had a severe case of athlete's foot since last month. The itching is driving me crazy. I can't take it anymore.

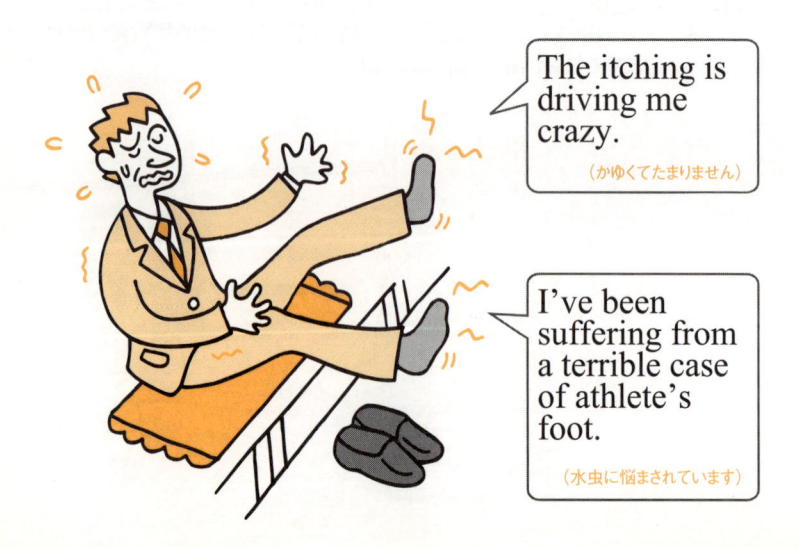

The itching is driving me crazy.
（かゆくてたまりません）

I've been suffering from a terrible case of athlete's foot.
（水虫に悩まされています）

Chapter 9 皮膚科での英会話

3 ドクター田中

診せてください。

Please show me.

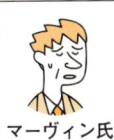

4 マーヴィン氏

はい。

Sure.

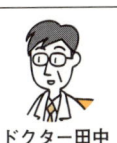

5 ドクター田中

ひどいようですね。軟膏をお出ししますから、患部につけてください。かゆみがとれても塗り続けてください。それから、足、特に指の間を乾かすように、通気性のよい靴を履き、同じ靴を毎日履かないこと。足が湿るようなら靴下を1日2度履き替えてください。

It's rather bad. I'll give you some ointment to apply on the fungus infected area. Do not discontinue even if the itchiness disappears. And, keep your feet dry, particularly the area between your toes. Wear well-ventilated shoes and do not wear the same shoes every day. Change your socks twice a day if your feet sweat a lot.

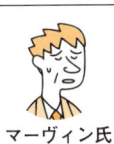

6 マーヴィン氏

わかりました。

All right.

皮膚科用語

あか

あかぎれ	cracks, chaps
痣	birthmark
あせも	heat rash
いぼ	wart, verruca
膿	pus
かゆみ	itching sensation, itchiness
抗ヒスタミン剤	antihistamine

さたな

しもやけ	chilblain, frostbite
消毒	disinfection
食物アレルギー	food allergies
じんま疹	hives
水疱	blister
帯状疱疹	herpes zoster
軟膏	ointment
にきび	acne

は

腫れ物	swelling
皮膚炎	dermatitis
日焼け	sunburn
発疹	rash

まやらわ

水虫	athlete's foot
虫刺され	insect bites
薬疹	drug eruption
薬物アレルギー	drug allergies
やけど	burn
レーザー手術	laser surgery
わきが、体臭	body odor

ちょっと一言 Medi Talk まとめ

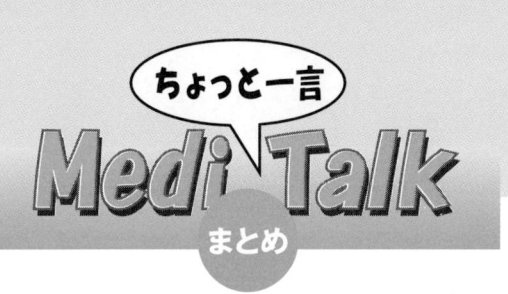

髙階: 外来や病棟に限らず、ナースの方々はドクターの方々よりも、患者さんと接する機会が多いのです。アメリカでは「ナース・プラクティショナー」の役割は大きく、都会から離れた地域では、近くにドクターがいないような場合が多いため、いちばん頼りになるのはこのナース・プラクティショナーなのです。
宮崎: そうですね。
髙階: 彼らの仕事の内容は、患者さんとの面接から始まり、急患に対する一般的な診察や、ある程度の臨床診断を行うことができ、また緊急時の静脈注射も許可されていますから、臨床の第一線では非常に大きな存在です。
宮崎: アメリカと日本では、まだまだ医療事情に差があるようですね。
髙階: 将来、わが国の医療もこのような形になっていくと思われますので、この際、患者さんの問診を行ったり、聴診を行ったりすることは、ドクターだけの仕事だと思わないでいただきたいと思います。臨床の現場では、何といってもチーム医療が大切なのです。少しでも早く患者さんの訴えを聞き、適切に対処することが求められているのです。
では、ここですでに出てきた会話もありますが、そのほかの系統歴をどう聞けばよいかについて、もう一度、練習をかねて次の会話を聞いてみましょう。

＊頭部(head)
● 頭蓋にけがをしたり、腫瘤ができたことはありますか？
Have you ever had any injury or abnormal mass in your skull?

● 今までに意識を失ったことがありますか？
Have you ever lost consciousness?

ちょっと一言 Medi Talk

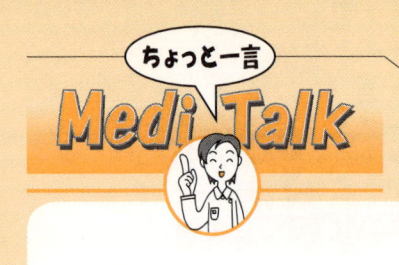

- 手や脚にしびれがありますか？

  Do you feel numbness in your hands or legs?

*頸部 (neck)
- 今までに主治医の先生から、甲状腺に異常があると言われたことがありますか？

  Have you ever been told by your doctor that you had thyroid trouble?

- 自分で、頸部の腫れに気付いたことがありますか？

  Have you ever noticed a swelling in your neck?

*乳房 (breasts)
- 乳房にしこりができたことがありますか？

  Have you had any lumps in your breasts?

- お子さんは母乳栄養ですか？　何か問題はありましたか？

  Did you breast-feed your children? Was there any problem?

*消化器 (gastrointestinal system)
- 食欲はありますか？

  Do you have a good appetite?

ちょっと一言 Medi Talk

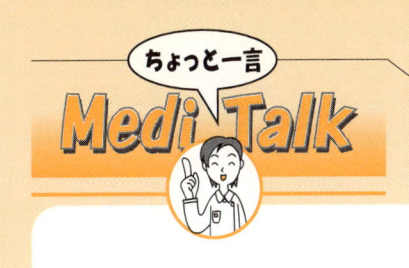

●消化不良を起こしたことがありますか？ もしあれば、どんな時ですか？
Do you have indigestion, and if so, when?

●むかつきを起こしたり、ときどき吐き気を催したりしますか？
Do you feel nauseated or vomit sometimes?

●どんな食べ物がお好きですか？
What kind of food do you like?

●黄疸にかかったことがありますか？
Have you ever had a jaundice?

●腹部に痛みや、塊ができたり、お腹の大きさが変わったことがありますか？
Have you had any pain, mass or change in size of your abdomen before?

●便通はどうですか？ 毎日便通がありますか？
How about your bowel habits? Do you have a bowel movement everyday?

ちょっと一言 Medi Talk

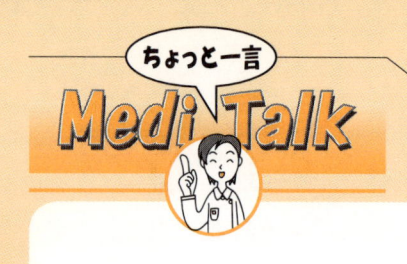

- 大便はどんな色ですか？　最近、色が変わったことに気付きましたか？

  What color is your stool? Have you noticed any change in the color recently?

- よく便秘しますか？

  Are you constipated frequently?

- 大便に血が混ざったことがありますか？

  Have you had any blood in your stool?

*泌尿器 (urology)

- 毎日、何回小便に行きますか？

  How many times do you pass urine everyday?

- 夜中にトイレに行きますか？

  Do you have to get up at night to urinate?

- 尿に膿が混じっていたことがありますか？

  Have you noticed any pus in your urine?

- 尿に糖が出ることがありますか？

  Do you have any sugar in your urine?

ちょっと一言 Medi Talk

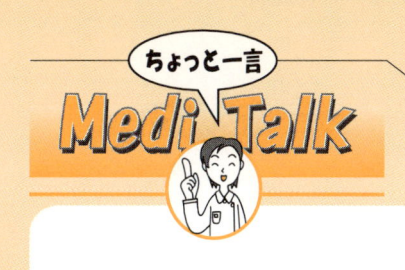

●主治医の先生から、尿に蛋白が出ていると言われたことがありますか？

Has it been pointed out by your doctor that you have albumin in your urine?

●排尿するのに力んだり、尿が出る前に少し時間がかかりますか？

Do you have to strain to urinate, or do you have to wait a little before urinating?

●尿線が細くなったり、途切れたりしたのに気付いたことがありますか？

Have you noticed any change in the size or force of stream of your urine?

●排尿の際に痛みを感じますか？

Do you feel any pain when you urinate?

＊婦人科 (gynecology)

●痛みなしに性交ができますか？

Are you able to have sexual intercourse without difficulty?

●生理は順調ですか？

How about your periods. Are they regular?

ちょっと一言 Medi Talk

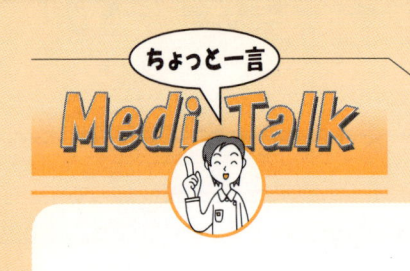

● 生理が始まったのは何歳の時ですか？
At what age did you begin to menstruate?

● 毎回、量が多いですか？
Do you have much flow each time?

● 1日にいくつパッドを使いますか？
How many pads do you have to use a day?

● 最終月経はいつでしたか？
When was your last menstrual period?

● お子さんは何人ですか？
How many children do you have?

● 最後のお産はいつでしたか？
When was your last delivery?

● 分娩の際、合併症を起こしましたか？
Did you have any complications with your deliveries?

Medi Talk ちょっと一言

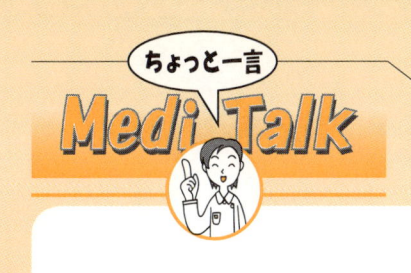

*性病 (venereal disease)

● 生理の間に性器出血やおりものがありますか？
Do you have any vaginal bleeding or discharge between your periods?

● 性病にかかったことはありますか？
Have you ever had a venereal disease?

● いちばん最近の性交はいつでしたか？
When was your last contact (sexual intercourse)?

● エイズの血液検査を受けたことがありますか？
Have you ever received a blood test for HIV (AIDS)?

● 最後の血清梅毒反応検査の結果はどうでしたか？
What was the result of your last serology test?

● 梅毒が陰性である血液検査の報告書をお持ちですか？
Do you have a report to show that the blood test was negative for syphilis?

ちょっと一言 Medi Talk

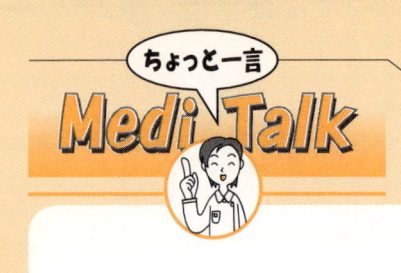

*神経筋肉系 (neuromuscular system)
● どこか筋肉の麻痺や、筋力の低下に気付いたことがありますか？

Do you have any muscular paralysis, or have you noticed any muscle weakness?

● 意識を失ったり、失神しそうになったことがありますか？

Have you ever lost consciousness or fainted?

● けいれんを起こしたことがありますか？

Have you ever had a convulsion (seizure)?

● 原因がわからずにバランスを失ったことがありますか？

Have you ever lost your balance without knowing the cause?

● 脳神経外科医や、精神科医に診てもらったことがありますか？

Have you ever consulted a neurosurgeon or psychiatrist?

*骨格系 (skeletal system)
● 関節痛や関節の運動制限を起こしたことがありますか？

Have you had any joint pains or limited motion?

ちょっと一言 Medi Talk

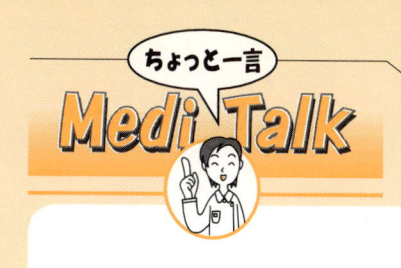

● 最近、体重の増減はありませんか？
Have you lost or gained weight recently?

＊与薬の説明 (explanation of how to take medicine)

● これは坐薬です。
This is a suppository.

● 高熱が続く時には、これを肛門に挿入してください。
Please insert it into your anus, when you suffer from continuous high fever.

● 痛みのある時に
in case you have pain

● 1回1錠／1カプセル
one pill / one capsule

● 6時間以上
over 6 hours

● 1日1回
once a day

● 1日2回
twice a day

ちょっと一言 Medi Talk

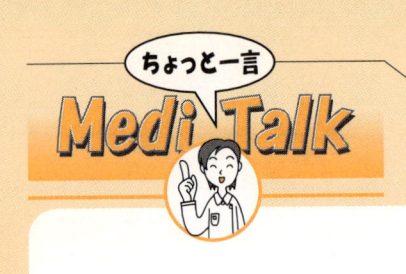

- 1日3回
three times a day

- 1日4回
four times a day

- 6時間ごと
every 6 hours

- かゆい時
when it is itching

- 痛む時
when you have pain

- 毎食前（後）
before (after) each meal

- 就寝前・朝食前・昼食前・夕食前・食前
before: bedtime, breakfast, lunch, dinner, eating

- 食間
between meals

- この錠剤を1日3回10日間飲んでください。
take these pills three times a day for ten days.

ちょっと一言 Medi Talk

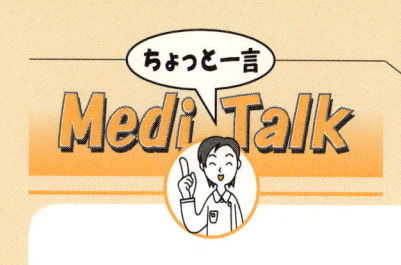

● 6時間ごとに坐薬を使ってください。
Use a suppository every 6 hours.

● この薬は頓服です。
This is a special medicine, for when you really need it.

● このお薬は少し眠くなるかもしれません。
This medicine will make you a little sleepy.

● できれば、ミルクと一緒に服用しないでください。
You had better not take it with milk.

● 粉薬は服用できますか。
Can you take powder medicine?

● お薬は忘れずに服用していますか。
Do you take the medicine regularly?

● では、お大事に。
Take it easy, please.

系統歴

あ

温かい	warm
荒れている	coarse
易疲感	easy fatigability
運動制限	limitation of motion
嚥下困難	difficulty of swallowing, dysphagia
黄疸	jaundice
悪寒	chills
おでき	boil(s)

か

咳嗽	cough
喀痰	sputum, phlegm, expectorate
肩の痛み	pain in shoulders
肩のこり	stiffness of shoulders
眼球充血	red eyes, hyperemia of conjunctive
眼球痛	pain in eye(s)
乾燥	dry
胸痛	chest pain, pain in chest
頸部硬直	stiffness of neck, nuchal rigidity
頸部腫脹	swelling of neck
頸部の拍動	pulsation of neck
幻覚	hallucination
健忘症	forgetfulness
口渇	excessive thirst
口臭	bad breath, foul mouth
口唇のけいれん	twitching of lips
紅潮	flush
口内痛	sore mouth
声の変化	change in voice

さ

嗄声	hoarseness
湿度	moisture

	歯肉痛	sore gums
	食欲不振	poor appetite, anorexia
	心悸亢進	palpitations
	心臓部痛	precordial pain, pain in the region of the heart
	頭軽感	light headedness
	頭重感	heaviness in head
	頭痛	headache
	舌苔	coated tongue, tongue membrane
	全身けいれん	convulsion(s)
	全身症状	general conditions (symptoms)
	喘鳴	wheezing
	蒼白	pallor
た	冷たい	cold
な	難聴	hearing trouble
	乳頭の分泌物	nipple discharge
	乳房腫瘤	lump in breast
	乳房疼痛	painful breasts
	熱性疱疹	fever blister(s)
は	発汗	sweating, sweat, perspiration
	発熱	fever
	鼻汁	discharge from nose, rhinorrhea
	鼻出血	bleeding from nose, epistaxis
	皮膚の色	color of skin
	皮膚の温度	temperature of skin
	皮膚の状態	skin texture
	皮膚の弾力性	elasticity
	皮膚病	skin disease, dermatosis

	鼻閉塞	nasal obstruction, stopped-up nose
	不安状態	anxiety
ま	味覚の変化	change of taste
	耳鳴り	ringing in ear, tinnitus
	耳の外傷	injury to ear
	無意識	unconsciousness
	めまい	dizziness, vertigo
	盲点	blind spot(s)
	毛髪の疾患	hair disease
や	抑うつ状態	depression
ら	流涎	salivation
	流涙	tearing, watering of the eye (lacrimation)
	リンパ節腫脹	swollen glands

系統歴の取り方

一般	過去3か月の体重の変化	weight change in last 3 months
	虚弱、無力	weakness
	疲労	fatigue
	悪寒	chills
	発汗	sweating

皮膚	発疹	rash
	かゆみ	itching
	爪の変化	nail changes

眼	視力の変化	vision problems
	眼鏡	glasses
	複視、二重視	diplopia
	光恐怖（光過敏、光痛）	photophobia
	炎症	inflammation
	痛み	pain
	ぼやける	blurring

耳	痛み	pain
	聴覚障害、難聴	deafness
	分泌物	discharges
	耳鳴り	tinnitus
	めまい	vertigo

鼻・咽喉	副鼻腔炎	sinusitis
	鼻出血	epistaxis
	歯の障害	teeth problems
	咽喉の痛み	sore throat
	かすれ声	hoarseness

呼吸器

喘鳴	wheezing
呼吸困難	dyspnea
胸膜の痛み	pleuritic pain
咳	cough
痰	sputum
喀血	hemoptysis
ツベルクリン	tuberculin
精製ツベルクリン	purified protein delivative (PPD)
接種日	inoculation date
結果	result

乳房

腫瘍	lumps
痛み	pain
分泌物	discharge
乳頭の変化	nipple change
マンモグラフィー	mammography

循環器

動悸	palpitation
痛み	pain
雑音	murmur
高/低 血圧	high/low BP (blood pressure)
跛行	claudication
疲労	fatigue
呼吸困難	dyspnea
起坐呼吸	orthopnea
発作性夜間呼吸困難	PND (paroxysmal nocternal dyspnea)
夜間多尿	nocturnal polyuria
浮腫	edema

消化器

食欲の変化	appetite change
嚥下困難	swallowing difficulty

	消化不良	indigestion
	ガス	gas
	吐き気	nausea
	嘔吐	vomiting
	吐血	hematemesis
	痛み	pain
	黄疸	jaundice
	ヘルニア	hernias
	メレナ（黒色タール便）	melena, tarry stool
	便秘	constipation
	緩下薬の使用	laxative use
	下痢	diarrhea
	痔	hemorrhoids
	便通の変化	change in bowel movement
尿生殖器	排尿障害	dysuria
	頻度	frequency
	尿意促迫	urgency
	失禁	incontinence
	血尿	hematuria
	夜間多尿	nocturnal polyuria
	側腹部痛	flank pain
	陰茎からの分泌	penile discharge
	前立腺の検査	prostate examination
血液	貧血	anemia
	リンパ節肥大	lymph node enlargement
	出血	bleeding
内分泌	糖尿病	diabetes mellitus
	甲状腺腫	goiter

アレルギー		
	湿疹	eczema
	喘息	asthma
	花粉症	hay fever
	じんま疹	hives

筋肉・骨格		
	外傷	trauma
	腫脹	swelling
	痛み	pain
	関節炎	arthritis
	関節可動域	full ROM (range of motion)

神経		
	失神	syncope
	発作	seizures
	麻痺	paralysis
	歩行障害	gait disorder
	協調	coordination
	感覚	sensation

精神		
	記憶	memory
	気分	mood
	不安	anxiety
	睡眠パターン	sleep pattern
	感情障害	emotional disturbance

性行動		
	性行為	sexual activity
	性欲の変化	libido change
	異性愛者	heterosexual
	同性/両性愛者	homosexual / bisexual
	特定の一人との性行為	single sexual partner
	複数との性行為	multiple sexual partner
	不妊	sterility
	不能	impotence

	性感染病	STD (sexually transmitted disease)
産婦人科	避妊薬	contraception
	初潮	menarche
	周期 / 期間 / 量	cycle / duration / amount
	規則性	regularity
	月経困難症	dysmenorrhea
	少量の出血	spotting
	分泌物	discharge
	閉経	menopause
	骨盤の検査	pelvic examination
	パパニコロー染色	PAP smear
	妊婦	gravida
	経産婦	para
	流産	abortions
	家庭内暴力の被害	victim of domestic violence
老年医学 (65歳以上)	認知障害	cognitive impairment
	抑うつ	depression
	転倒 / 事故	falls / accidents
	失禁	incontinence
予防接種	インフルエンザ接種	flu vaccine
	破傷風	tetanus
	ジフテリア	diphtheria
	A型肝炎	hepatitis A
	B型肝炎	hepatitis B

体を表す用語

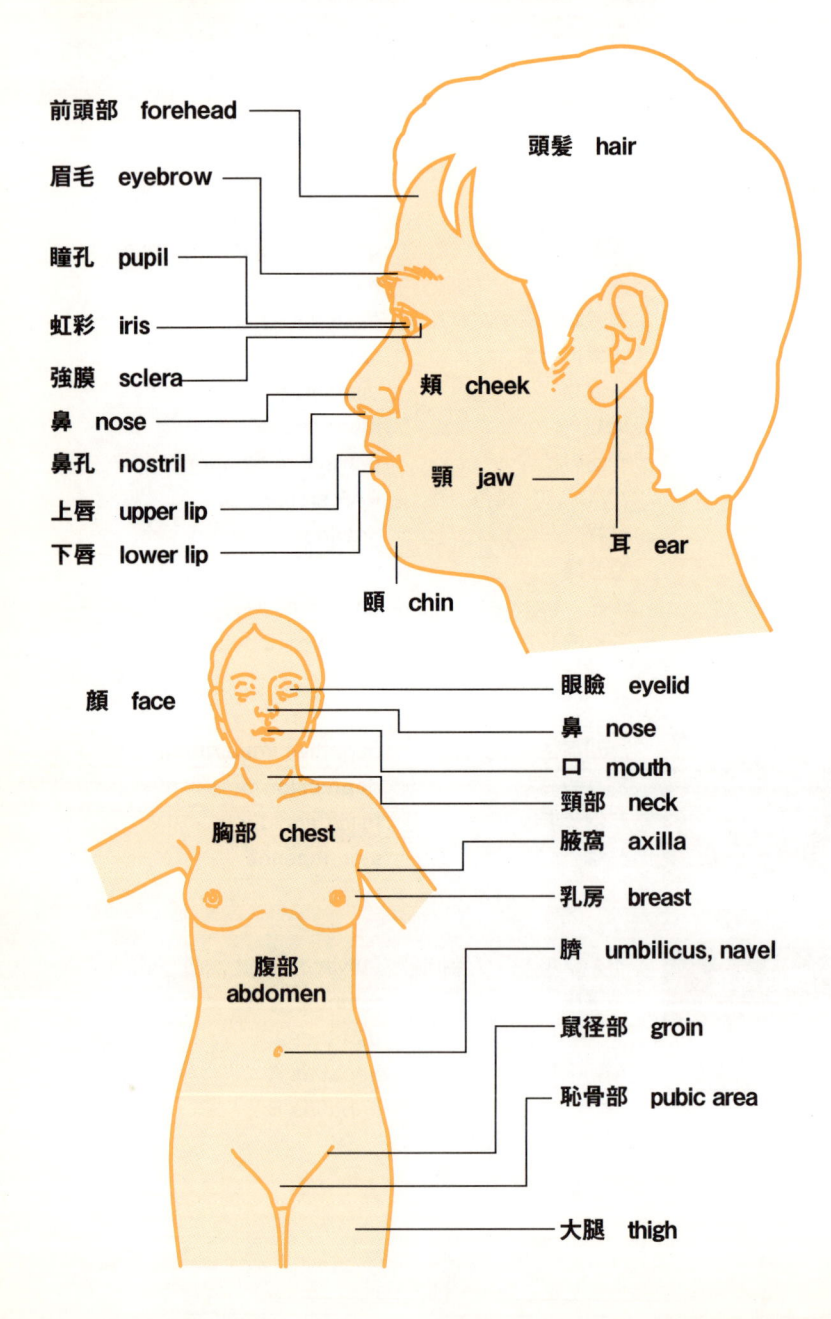

前頭部	forehead
眉毛	eyebrow
瞳孔	pupil
虹彩	iris
強膜	sclera
鼻	nose
鼻孔	nostril
上唇	upper lip
下唇	lower lip
頭髪	hair
頬	cheek
顎	jaw
耳	ear
頤	chin
顔	face
眼瞼	eyelid
鼻	nose
口	mouth
頸部	neck
腋窩	axilla
胸部	chest
乳房	breast
腹部	abdomen
臍	umbilicus, navel
鼠径部	groin
恥骨部	pubic area
大腿	thigh

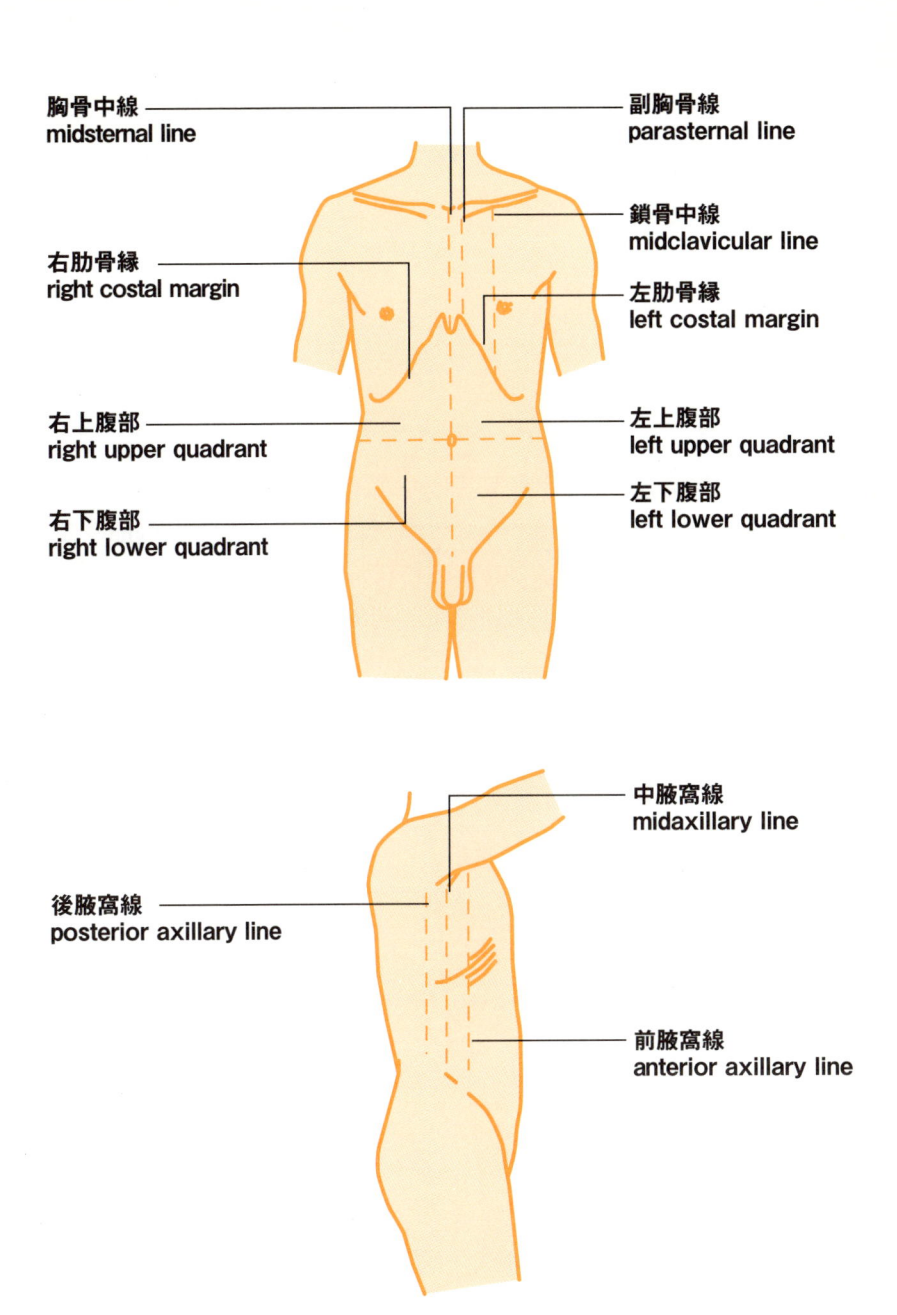

胸骨中線	midsternal line
副胸骨線	parasternal line
鎖骨中線	midclavicular line
右肋骨縁	right costal margin
左肋骨縁	left costal margin
右上腹部	right upper quadrant
左上腹部	left upper quadrant
右下腹部	right lower quadrant
左下腹部	left lower quadrant
中腋窩線	midaxillary line
後腋窩線	posterior axillary line
前腋窩線	anterior axillary line

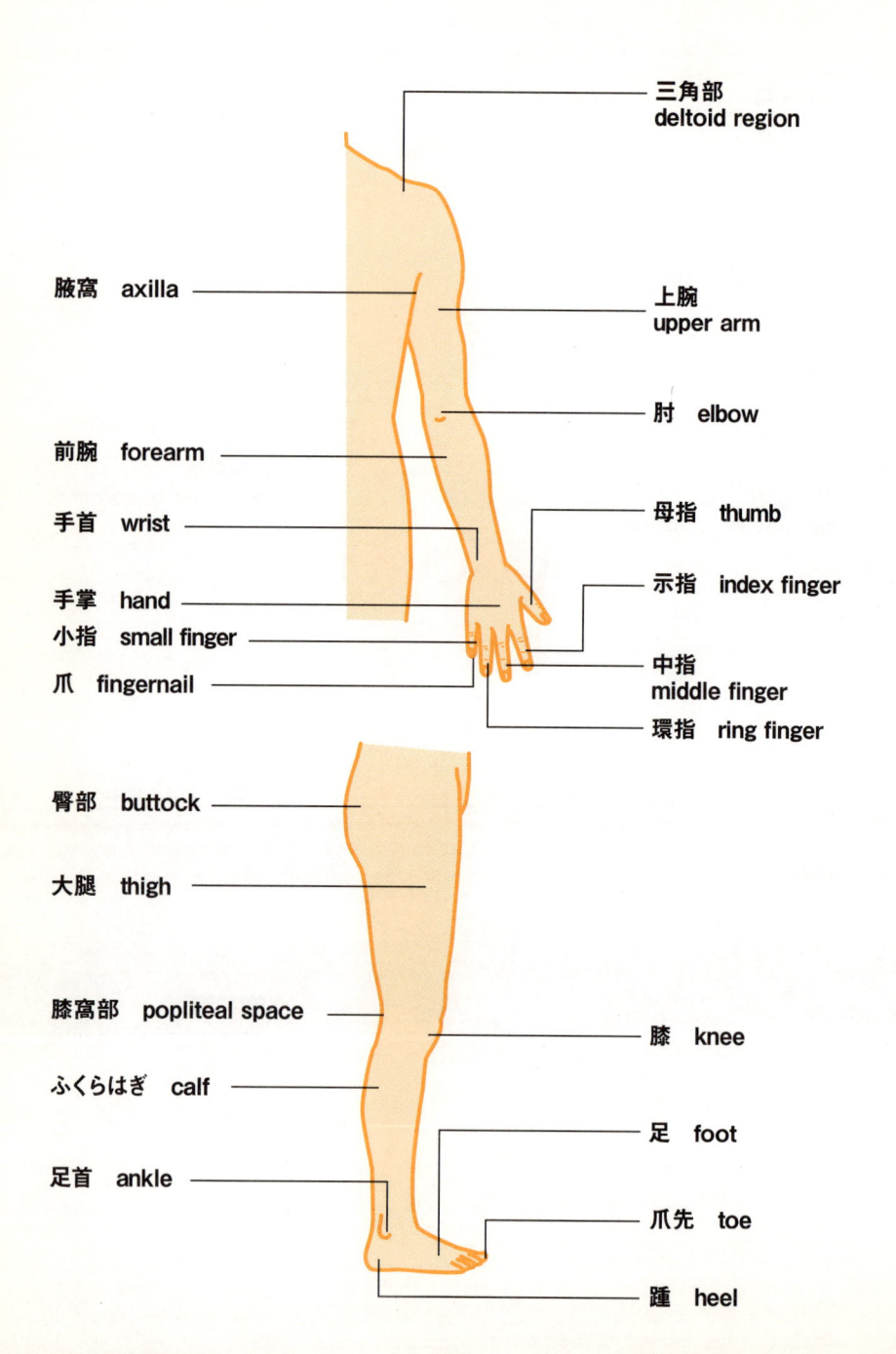

三角部	deltoid region
腋窩	axilla
上腕	upper arm
肘	elbow
前腕	forearm
手首	wrist
母指	thumb
手掌	hand
示指	index finger
小指	small finger
中指	middle finger
爪	fingernail
環指	ring finger
臀部	buttock
大腿	thigh
膝窩部	popliteal space
膝	knee
ふくらはぎ	calf
足	foot
足首	ankle
爪先	toe
踵	heel

著者・英文監修者プロフィール

【著者】
髙階經和(たかしな・つねかず)

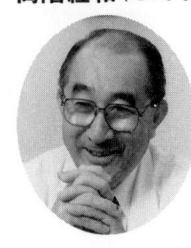

1929年	大阪府生まれ
1954年	神戸医科大学(現神戸大学医学部)卒業
1958年	米国チュレーン大学医学部留学
1962年	淀川キリスト教病院循環器科科長
1969年	髙階クリニック(現髙階国際クリニック)開設
	神戸大学医学部講師(医学英語・臨床心臓病学)
	(〜1985年)
1985年	大阪大学歯学部講師(歯科麻酔科)
	社団法人臨床心臓病学教育研究会会長

その間、チュレーン大学医学部、マイアミ大学医学部、および、アリゾナ大学医学部の客員教授を歴任。

医師のための英会話(鳳鳴堂書店)
心電図を学ぶ人のために(医学書院)
看護英会話のライセンス(医学書院)
医学英会話のライセンス(医学書院)
国際医学会のための実践英会話(南江堂)
CDで学ぶ実践診療英会話(南江堂)
やってみようよ! 心電図(インターメディカ)
続・やってみようよ! 心電図(インターメディカ) ほか著書多数
発表論文では、英語論文:38編、日本語論文:225編

【著者】
宮崎悦子(みやざき・えつこ)

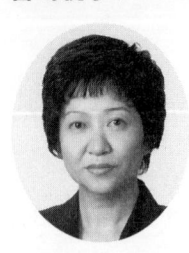

1956年	大阪府生まれ
1979年	京都外国語大学イスパニア語学科卒業
1981年	髙階クリニック(現髙階国際クリニック)秘書勤務
	(〜1983年)
1994年	社団法人臨床心臓病学教育研究会事務局勤務
	外国人医療相談活動にボランティアとして参加。その間、日英対訳の小冊子「MEDITALK」シリーズの編集・制作を手掛ける。

【英文監修】
テレンス ジェイムズ オブライエン（テリー オブライエン）

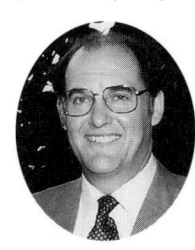

1948年　シェフィールド、イギリス生まれ
1967年　シェフィールド美術大学
1968年　カーディフ美術大学学士号取得
1971年　ブライトン　ポリテクニック大学　美術教員免許取得
1995年　リーズ大学大学院　TESOL
1978年　大谷女子大学非常勤
1980年　大谷女子大学講師
1985年　大谷女子大学助教授
1993年　大谷女子大学教授

著書に
Essays on Teaching English as a Second Language（アポロン社）
Clearly Britain, Clearly Japan（南雲堂）
A Trip to Britain（南雲堂）
Looking Around England（南雲堂）
Bridge to College English（南雲堂）
Spotlight on Britain（南雲堂）
などがある。

参考図書

1) 髙階經和, E.N.メルダール監修：医師のための英会話・全2巻, 鳳鳴堂書店, 1970.

2) 髙階經和：医学英会話のライセンス, 医学書院, 1975.

3) 髙階經和, 木下佳代子, G.Barraclough 英文監修：看護英会話のライセンス（第3版）, 医学書院, 1990.

4) 髙階經和：CDで学ぶ実践診療英会話, 南江堂, 1993.

5) 髙階經和, 梅田幸久, 永田登志子, 萬代隆, 宮崎悦子, テレンス・J・オブライエン英文監修：MEDITALK I, 社団法人臨床心臓病学教育研究会, 1995.

6) 髙階經和, 梅田幸久, 永田登志子, 萬代隆, 宮崎悦子, テレンス・J・オブライエン英文監修：MEDITALK II, 社団法人臨床心臓病学教育研究会, 1996.

7) 髙階經和, 梅田幸久, 永田登志子, 萬代隆, 宮崎悦子, テレンス・J・オブライエン英文監修：MEDITALK III, 社団法人臨床心臓病学教育研究会, 1998.

ちょっと一言　MediTalk
医療現場で役立つ英会話

2005年3月10日　初版第1刷発行

- ［著　　者］髙階經和・宮崎悦子
- ［英文監修］テレンス ジェイムズ オブライエン
- ［発 行 者］赤土正幸
- ［発 行 所］株式会社インターメディカ
  　　　　　〒102-0072
  　　　　　東京都千代田区飯田橋2-14-2
  　　　　　TEL　03-3234-9559
  　　　　　FAX　03-3239-3066
  　　　　　URL　http://www.intermedica.co.jp
- ［印　　刷］凸版印刷株式会社

編集／小沢ひとみ
デザイン／安藤千恵（AS）
DTP／ブルーインク
イラスト／松田健
ISBN 4-89996-116-2 C3047
定価はカバーに表示してあります。